1990

Restructuring for Ambulatory Care

A Guide to Reorganization

Edited by Theodore A. Matson
*Division of Ambulatory Care and Health Promotion
of the American Hospital Association*

AHA®

American Hospital Publishing, Inc.,
a wholly owned subsidiary of the
American Hospital Association

The views expressed in this publication are strictly those of the authors and do not necessarily represent official positions of the American Hospital Association.

Library of Congress Cataloging-in-Publication Data

Restructuring for ambulatory care : a guide to reorganization / edited by
    Theodore A. Matson.
             p.   cm.
        Includes bibliographical references.
        ISBN 1-55648-045-8
        1. Hospitals—Outpatient services—Administration.
  2. Ambulatory medical care—Administration. I. Matson, Theodore A.
    [DNLM: 1. Ambulatory Care—economics—United States.
  2. Ambulatory Care—organization & administration—United States.
  3. Ambulatory Care—trends—United States. 4. Ambulatory Care
  Facilities—United States. 5. Hospital Administration—United
  States.   WX 205 R436]
  RA974.R47   1990
  362.1'2—dc20
  DNLM/DLC   89-18507
  for Library of Congress   CIP

Catalog no. 016143

©1990 by American Hospital Publishing, Inc.,
a wholly owned subsidiary of the
American Hospital Association

Printed in the USA

Text set in English Times
2.5M—02/90—0253

Marlene Chamberlain, Project Editor
Linda Conheady, Manuscript Editor
Lawrence Denne, Editorial Assistant
Marcia Bottoms, Managing Editor
Peggy DuMais, Production Coordinator
Marcia Vecchione, Designer
Brian Schenk, Books Division Director

Contents

List of Figures

List of Tables

Contributors

Thomas P. Berry, A.I.A, is vice-president for business development, Marshall Erdman and Associates, Madison, Wisconsin. Mr. Berry is actively involved in all major ambulatory care projects including hospital-based medical office buildings, integrated physicians' office buildings, ambulatory care centers on hospital campuses, and large multispecialty group practice facilities. Mr. Berry is a frequent lecturer for the MGMA, FASA, and AHA-SACP. He is also a member of the Society for Ambulatory Care Professionals.

Sister Elise Boudreaux, D.C., M.S.N., is president, Providence Medical Center, Mobile, Alabama. She is also a member of the American College of Healthcare Executives and a member of the Alabama Association of Hospital Executives. Her previous experience includes numerous nursing management and administrative positions within the Daughters of Charity of St. Vincent de Paul health system. She served 12 years as president of the East Central Province of the Daughters of Charity at the Evansville, Indiana, corporate office, overseeing the health care ministry activities of nine central states.

Alice D'Alessio is director of communications, Marshall Erdman and Associates, Inc., Madison, Wisconsin, with responsibility for analyzing and reporting in the areas of health care design and construction and preparing policy papers and informational literature. She has an extensive record of publication in the health care and environmental fields. For a number of years she authored a column on recent medical advances for *Madison Magazine* and in 1988 was editor of the guidebook *Organizing, Designing and Building Ambulatory Healthcare Facilities,* published by Marshall Erdman and Associates, Inc.

Richard B. Donker, Ph.D., is vice-president, clinical services, Memorial Hospitals Association; executive director, MediPLUS Health Plans, Inc.; and president, California Aeromedical Rescue and Evacuation, Inc. He currently has responsibility for all nonnursing unit clinical areas of Memorial Hospitals Association and directs the managed care contracting department. He also functions as executive director of a 4-hospital, 330-physician PPO corporation, and as president of a 3-hospital air-ambulance operation. Mr. Donker's 11 years with Memorial have included various management and planning functions. Among these were development and initial management of Memorial's helicopter ambulance, PromptCare urgent care centers, Health PLUS employee assistance program and wellness programs, sports medicine and occupational care center, employee health system, seniors' program, and managed care contracting department.

William J. Graham, M.B.A., is principal, Bill Graham & Associates, Colorado Springs, Colorado. Bill Graham established Bill Graham & Associates after ten years of experience as the senior marketing officer for several large hospitals and diversified health care systems. Mr. Graham's experience includes managing strategic planning, market research, new business development, joint ventures, and physician bonding programs, as well as developing and managing marketing communications. As vice-president for marketing services for Penrose Health System, Colorado Springs, Colorado, a highly diversified operator of two hospitals, ambulatory care and urgent care centers, a PPO, and other joint ventures, he engineered several campaigns that reversed a five-year decline in market share. He is on the board of directors for the Academy of Health Services Marketing and is a frequent speaker and writer on strategic marketing management in health care.

Diane M. Howard, M.P.H., is director, Division of Ambulatory Care and Health Promotion, American Hospital Association, Chicago, Illinois. As division director, she is responsible for providing representation, advocacy, and membership services and for coordinating research and data in the areas of primary care, group practices, health maintenance organizations, ambulatory surgery, emergency medical services, freestanding urgent care centers, home care, hospice, and corporate and personal health programming. In addition, she coordinates educational services to AHA membership, acts as director of the Society for Ambulatory Care Professionals, and participates in policy development. She is currently assistant professor, Department of Health Systems Management, College of Health Sciences, Rush University, Chicago, Illinois. She is a national speaker in the areas of ambulatory care and hospital diversification and has published many articles. She is also the editor of *New Business Development in Ambulatory Care: Exploring Diversification Options,* published by American Hospital Publishing, Inc.

James A. Lamb, M.H.A., is president and chairman of the board of Washoe Health System, Inc., Reno, Nevada, parent company of Washoe Medical Center, Inc. Mr. Lamb is also president and chief executive officer of the medical center. For 14 years, he was a member of the management staff of Baroness Erlanger and T. C. Thompson Children's Hospitals in Chattanooga, Tennessee. For 9 years, Mr. Lamb was president and chief executive officer of the Chattanooga Hamilton County Hospital Authority, the owner and governing body of Erlanger and Children's Hospitals. In 1983, he was appointed chief executive officer of Washoe Medical Center. The medical center reorganized in 1985 into a health care system and Mr. Lamb was appointed to his current position. He is a member of the American College of Health Care Executives and is on the advisory committee of the American Hospital Association's Division of Ambulatory Care. He also serves as an alternate delegate to the Regional Advisory Board, Region IX, of the American Hospital Association.

Douglas M. Mancino, J.D., is partner, McDermott, Will & Emery, Los Angeles, California. Mr. Mancino has extensive experience representing hospitals, health care organizations, and physicians in the development and operation of ambulatory care programs such as surgery centers, imaging centers, freestanding cancer centers, and similar fixed and mobile ambulatory care delivery systems. Mr. Mancino is coauthor of *Joint Ventures Between Hospitals and Physicians* (Aspen Systems Corp., 1987), has authored numerous articles and book chapters on various topics pertaining to ambulatory care, and is a frequent speaker on legal and business issues affecting hospital and health care providers. Mr. Mancino is a member of the board of directors of the American Academy of Hospital Attorneys and is a member of the Tax Advisory Group of the American Hospital Association's Office of Legal and Regulatory Affairs. Mr. Mancino serves on the editorial advisory board of *Decisions in Technology Economics,* a publication of GE Medical Systems.

Ellen Marszalek-Gaucher, M.S., is senior associate director, University of Michigan Hospitals, Ann Arbor, Michigan. She manages the operation of an 888-bed hospital with 32,000 admissions per year and 780,000 outpatient clinic visits. She serves on the editorial board of *Health Care Competition* newsletter and the executive committee of the National Demonstration Project on Quality funded by the Hartford Foundation and the Harvard Community Health Plan. She is a member of the American College for Health Care Executives and a charter member of the Society for Ambulatory Care Professionals. She is coauthoring a book called *Transforming Healthcare Organization* for Jossey-Bass Publishers. Previously she was the associate director of ambulatory care and played a major role in the design and activation of the A. Alfred Taubman Center, a 300,000-square-foot ambulatory care center. She also developed plans and implemented a satellite network of six comprehensive primary care centers and three specialty clinics.

William C. Mason, M.H.A., is president and chief executive officer, Baptist Health, Inc., Jacksonville, Florida. He is president and chief executive officer of Baptist Medical Center, a 579-bed tertiary care hospital, Baptist Health Foundation, a philanthropic organization, and Healthcare Management Services, Inc., a subsidiary for-profit corporation of BHI. Prior to his service at Baptist Medical Center, his activities included service as chief executive officer of hospitals in Bangalore, India, and Tanzania, Africa. Mr. Mason also served as a foreign service officer with the U.S. Department of State in Manila, Philippine Islands, and Saigon, Vietnam, where he was assigned to host country ministries of health to develop hospitals and medical schools. He is a Fellow of the American College of Healthcare Executives.

Theodore A. Matson, M.A., is senior staff specialist, Division of Ambulatory Care and Health Promotion, American Hospital Association, Chicago, Illinois. In this capacity, he is responsible for providing strategic direction and consultation to the health care industry in the areas of hospital-based ambulatory care services, ambulatory surgery, freestanding ambulatory care facilities, and emergency medical services. In addition, he provides representation and advocacy services and participates in public policy developments regarding ambulatory care issues. Mr. Matson is a national and international speaker in ambulatory care. He serves as editor of the American Hospital Association's publication *Outreach,* the sole industry resource devoted exclusively to hospital perspectives on ambulatory care issues. A frequent writer on ambulatory care topics, he is also the editor of *The Hospital Emergency Department: Returning to Financial Viability,* published by American Hospital Publishing, Inc.

Kenneth J. Natzke, M.B.A., is administrator/chief executive officer, St. Joseph Hospital Medical Center, Bloomington, Illinois. He is a member of the multiinstitutional system of the Sisters of the Third Order of St. Francis, Peoria, Illinois.

Patrick W. Philbin, M.S.W., M.H.A., is president, Patrick Philbin & Associates, Austin, Texas. He is also chairman of the board of Physicians Development Resources and American Retirement Management. Patrick Philbin & Associates specializes in strategic planning, new era ambulatory care and health campus development, physician practice enhancement services, cost reduction programs, and management consultation. Mr. Philbin's experience spans all sides of the health care industry, including being part of administration at Henry Ford Hospital in Detroit, Michigan; doing corporate planning and marketing at St. Vincent Hospital and Healthcare Center in Indianapolis, Indiana; serving as associate director of the Metropolitan Health Board (HSA) in Minneapolis/St. Paul, Minnesota; being the administrator of a Michigan state juvenile detention center; and doing private practice in mental health therapy. He has served on numerous committees and speaks nationally on ambulatory care, the future of health care, management practices, and other relevant topics. He has published in several magazines.

Clarice V. Rech, R.N., M.P.A., is manager, Northwest Community Hospital Treatment Center, Buffalo Grove, Illinois. She developed and directed the implementation of an 11,000-square-foot treatment center. She has managed the ongoing operation since its inception. Buffalo Grove Treatment Center was noted as the busiest hospital-operated outpatient treatment center by the Metropolitan Chicago Healthcare Council in an article in *Chicago Consumer* magazine, July–August 1987. In an article entitled "The Experience Factor," Buffalo Grove Treatment Center was named number one, treating 32,501 patients annually.

Susan Strong is director of communication, Drexel Toland & Associates, Memphis, Tennessee, a consulting firm that specializes in medical office buildings, ambulatory care facilities, hospitals, and other related medical buildings. At DT&A she has contributed extensively to the company's pioneering development of studies in medical manpower analysis and medical staff master planning. She is coauthor of *Hospital-Based Medical Office Buildings,* published by American Hospital Publishing, Inc. A writer and editor for almost 25 years, she directed communication programs for such firms as Hospital Corporation of America, the Methodist Publishing House, Service Merchandise Company, and Kentucky Fried Chicken Corporation before joining Drexel Toland & Associates.

Drexel Toland, M.S.H.A., is president of Drexel Toland & Associates, Memphis, Tennessee; a Fellow of the American College of Healthcare Executives; and a nationally recognized authority on hospital-related medical office buildings and ambulatory care facilities. Since forming his consulting firm in 1968, he has advised over 225 clients in planning, designing, and constructing their hospital-based medical office buildings and ambulatory care and hospital facilities. His firm has designed suites for over 11,000 physicians and 10 million square feet of space. For 14 years he served as assistant administrator of the 2,000-bed Baptist Memorial Hospital, Memphis, Tennessee, the first hospital in the country to own and operate its own medical office building and hotel. It now has four office towers, three of which were built or acquired and managed under Mr. Toland's supervision. Mr. Toland coauthored the book *Hospital-Based Medical Office Buildings,* first published in 1981 with the revised edition published and released in 1986 by American Hospital Publishing, Inc.

Preface

As hospitals enter the 1990s and beyond, few will anticipate the true impact of ambulatory care as a major force in the total spectrum of health care delivery. Despite the fundamental restructuring of our industry, which has promoted economies of scale and lower costs for alternatives for care, an acute care mentality continues to exist — a philosophy that emphasizes that most hospital revenues will continue to come from inpatient services. It is often difficult to challenge this way of thinking, because on average 30 units of outpatient service are required to equal the revenue generated from a single inpatient admission. Furthermore, despite ambulatory care's phenomenal growth, profit margins associated with these services are small in relation to those of inpatient services.

Although many institutions continue to rely on the inpatient bed mentality, it is clear that the movement toward ambulatory care as the dominant line of business — now considered the new health care environment — is upon us all. In just four years, from 1983 to 1987, inpatient admissions to short-term community hospitals declined 10 percent while outpatient services soared in excess of 14 percent.[1]

This classic transformational shift from inpatients to outpatients is further illustrated by the revenues now represented in providing "core" ambulatory care services. In 1983, fewer than 12 percent of total hospital revenues resulted from outpatients; in 1987, 23 percent of total revenues were outpatient related — an increase of 92 percent.[2] Today, many hospitals that have successfully diversified in ambulatory care now report 40 to 60 percent of total revenues resulting from outpatients. By 1995, it is predicted that the majority of hospitals will experience a revenue mix of 50 percent inpatients and 50 percent outpatients.[3]

Overall, investing for the future in the new health care environment is a long-term rather than a short-term survival strategy. Because the reorganization and restructuring of health care is in its early stages, it is conceivable that the movement toward and domination of ambulatory care will continue for the next 20 years. To compete in this environment, hospitals must adopt a new philosophy, new priorities, and a new way of thinking about how services will be provided in cost-effective, delivery-efficient settings.

It is for these reasons that I have embarked upon this publishing effort. Having obtained administrative and operational ambulatory care experience in seven hospitals and at the American Hospital Association, I have developed a strong passion for the unique needs in ambulatory care environments. I truly hope that this publication will be of value to those seeking to create a competitive strategy for their ambulatory care services.

References

1. American Hospital Association. *Hospital Statistics,* 1984 and 1988 editions. Chicago: AHA, 1984 and 1988.

2. American Hospital Association.

3. Matson, T. A. The explosive growth of ambulatory care: challenges and opportunities for hospitals. Presentation, Evangelical Health Systems, Good Shepherd Hospital, Barrington, IL, Nov. 20, 1986.

Acknowledgments

I would like to offer my thanks to the many individuals who made this book a reality. First, to the contributors, all of whom were selected because of their knowledge and expertise. Thanks also to Cheryl Hardy, my secretary, who performed the monumental task of typing the manuscripts and seeing them to the production phase; to Ed Zimmerman, who provided invaluable market research that served as the cornerstone of my work; to Karen McGannon, senior project specialist, AHA Healthcare Administrative Services, who assisted me with infinite requests for utilization and financial data; to Marlene Chamberlain, product line manager, American Hospital Publishing, Inc., who provided a keen oversight of the manuscripts and the production process; to Linda Conheady, assistant managing editor, American Hospital Publishing, Inc., who provided excellent editorial assistance on the final manuscript; and to Brian Schenk, vice-president, Books Division, American Hospital Publishing, Inc., for his continued support of bringing state-of-the-art publications to the ambulatory care industry.

I would like to express appreciation to my colleagues in the Division of Ambulatory Care and Health Promotion for their encouragement and support and for the backup they provided when I worked on this endeavor. Many thanks to Maria Collier, Barbara Giloth, Lynn Jones, Dan Lerman, and Dorothy Wilson. Special thanks to Diane Howard for developing a very challenging work environment that fostered creativity and entrepreneurship and provided a chance to think and a place to grow. I feel fortunate, because many strive to find such an environment throughout their careers, but only a few find it.

Finally, I would like to thank my parents, both teachers and community leaders, who supported my ideas with as much thoughtfulness as they gave to their students and neighbors; and Mor Mor, my grandmother, who at 96 remains my most avid reader.

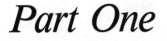

Part One

Creating a Competitive Edge

Chapter 1

An Industry Perspective

Theodore A. Matson and Patrick W. Philbin

Historically, ambulatory care has been provided by hospitals for various reasons: consumer demand for services; selective competition among hospitals and physicians; incentives from regulatory efforts of third-party payers, insurers, and regulators; responses to unmet service needs; and interest in teaching and research.

More recently, hospitals have expanded ambulatory care efforts in order to realize diversification and growth objectives, thus creating new markets for new as well as existing ambulatory care services.[1] Expansion has also occurred in order to maintain market share in areas where alternative delivery and financing entities, such as health maintenance organizations (HMOs) and preferred provider organizations (PPOs), have posed competitive threats. In addition, involvement by hospitals has accelerated because of the explosive growth of freestanding ambulatory competitors, namely, freestanding convenience clinics and surgery centers. To understand the significance of the expanding role of ambulatory care in the United States, it is appropriate to review the provision of services from a macro perspective.

Hospital-Based Ambulatory Care

Hospitals today are continuing to play a significant role in the provision of ambulatory care services. Currently, 4,242, or 67.5 percent, of the 6,281 hospitals have organized outpatient departments; 5,262, or 83.8 percent, of hospitals provide ambulatory surgical services; and 5,272, or 83.9 percent, of hospitals have emergency departments. Since the implementation of the Tax Equity and Fiscal Responsibility Act in 1983 and the prospective pricing system that promoted a competitive health care environment, ambulatory

3

care services have witnessed unprecedented growth. As shown in table 1-1, hospital-sponsored and -associated ambulatory care facilities provided 310.7 million services (physician visits, outpatient/ancillary services, and emergency department services) in 1987. This is an increase of 14.0 percent from 273.2 million services provided in 1983.

The numbers and types of ambulatory care programs and services have also increased substantially since 1983 (table 1-1). Most notably, health promotion services and home care programs have increased by 91 percent and 115 percent, respectively. Although traditional hospital-based ambulatory programs, such as emergency departments and office-based clinics, have long been established by hospitals, the broad expansion of ambulatory care services continues. According to a survey conducted by the American Hospital Association in 1986, ten ambulatory care programs were considered as targets for hospital diversification. Women's health services were ranked most frequently by hospitals (26 percent), followed by industrial/occupational medicine (19 percent), sports medicine (17 percent), health promotion (16 percent), home health (14 percent), diagnostic radiology (10 percent), ambulatory surgery (8 percent), diagnostic laboratory (7 percent), emergency services (4 percent), and physical therapy (4 percent).

Enhanced expansion of ambulatory care programs and services has resulted in a notable shifting of patient revenues from inpatient services to traditionally based ambulatory services. Revenues for ambulatory care services from all sources for short-term community hospitals were $37.2 billion in 1987, up from $11.7 billion in 1983. This represents an increase of $25.5 billion and is now equivalent to $126 per service, where service is defined to include the spectrum of visits and ancillary services. As a proportion of total hospital revenues, ambulatory services in 1987 accounted for 23 percent, with this projection increasing over time. Although outpatient revenues are small in comparison to total revenues, they are quite dramatic numerically.

As shown in figures 1-1 and 1-2, gross outpatient revenues have risen for hospitals in all bed-size categories and regions of the country. In terms of hospital bed size, the most prominent increases in outpatient revenues have occurred in facilities with 200 or fewer beds. These increases have occurred primarily because of the recent involvement of these facilities in various ambulatory care programs that previously were not provided or were underutilized. Outpatient revenues by regions of the country also yield interesting geographic trends. For instance, the Middle Atlantic, East North Central, East South Central, West North Central, and West South Central regions have posted in excess of 9 percent increases in revenue growth since 1983.

Clearly, the impact of hospital-sponsored ambulatory care services is changing the delivery structure of the traditional patient care process. Consequently, the ambulatory care industry has become a potent force in the

Table 1-1. Hospital-Sponsored Ambulatory Care Utilization Trends, 1983–1987

Number of Visits[a] (in thousands)	1983	1984	1985	1986	1987	Percentage Change 1983–1987
Ambulatory surgery[b]	4,987	5,827	7,308	8,705	9,757	96.0
Emergency department	77,522	78,492	80,079	82,117	83,478	8.0
Other outpatient[c]	195,646	198,074	202,060	212,516	227,229	23.0
Total outpatient visits[d]	273,168	276,566	282,139	294,633	310,707	14.0

Number of Hospital Programs[e]	1983	1984	1985	1986	1987	Percentage Change 1983–1987
Ambulatory surgery[f]	5,012	5,109	5,245	5,243	5,262	5.0
Emergency department	5,406	5,397	5,382	5,340	5,272	(3.0)
Organized outpatient department	3,021	3,191	3,434	3,989	4,242	47.0
Other outpatient:						
Health promotion	2,559	2,943	3,253	4,424	4,656	91.0
Home care	920	1,296	1,714	1,986	1,983	115.0
Hospice	548	616	727	827	820	48.0
Rehabilitation	2,146	2,248	2,398	2,329	2,443	20.0
Psychiatry	1,259	1,292	1,339	1,387	1,428	16.0
Chemical dependency	1,073	1,134	1,244	1,342	1,416	37.0

Source: Division of Ambulatory Care and Health Promotion, American Hospital Association.

[a]American Hospital Association's annual survey.

[b]Surgical services provided to patients who do not remain in the hospital overnight.

[c]Refers to outpatient therapy and treatment visits, ancillary service visits, and all other forms of outpatient care not previously defined; also includes ambulatory surgery visits.

[d]Visits by patients who are not lodged in the hospital while receiving medical, dental, or other services. Each appearance by an outpatient to each unit of the hospital counts as one outpatient visit. Total outpatient visits include emergency department and other outpatient visits; ambulatory surgery visits are included in the "other outpatient" visit category.

[e]American Hospital Association's *Hospital Statistics*; number of hospitals reporting for each year was approximately 90 percent.

[f]Information not reported until 1983.

Figure 1-1. Growth in Outpatient Revenue, by Hospital Bed Size, 1983–1987

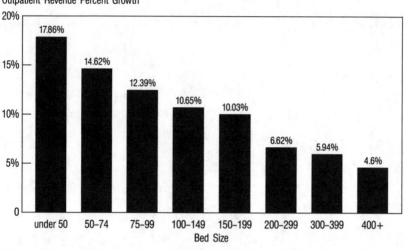

Outpatient Revenue Percent Growth

Source: HAS/MONITREND, American Hospital Association, 1987.

Figure 1-2. Growth in Outpatient Revenue, by Census Division, 1983–1987

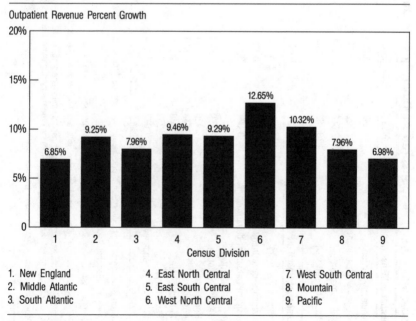

Outpatient Revenue Percent Growth

1. New England
2. Middle Atlantic
3. South Atlantic
4. East North Central
5. East South Central
6. West North Central
7. West South Central
8. Mountain
9. Pacific

Source: HAS/MONITREND, American Hospital Association, 1987.

health care marketplace. As the ambulatory care industry quickly evolves into a formidable player in this field, it will no doubt challenge the realities of the marketplace.

Freestanding Ambulatory Care

As hospitals have expanded their provision of ambulatory care services, complex and challenging environmental forces have led to widespread entrepreneurial activities in this arena; the result is that virtually all ambulatory care activities have evolved into multiple freestanding facilities. Today these freestanding alternatives have further challenged hospitals to provide ambulatory care services in cost-effective, delivery-efficient modes of operation. Although freestanding facilities command a small portion of utilization and revenues relative to hospitals, they have earned a significant and growing place in the health care marketplace. Freestanding facilities that provide urgent, episodic, and primary medical care, commonly referred to as convenience clinics, have increased from fewer than 300 facilities in 1980 to over 3,000 facilities in 1987, an increase of 400 percent. Further, it is estimated that 5,500 such facilities will be operational by 1990. In 1980, convenience clinics provided fewer than 5 million patient visits, compared to 43 million visits in 1987. Based upon year-to-year growth rates, patient visits to convenience clinics are estimated at 63 million by 1990.[2]

Despite their growth, freestanding convenience clinics have undergone tremendous change; only 30 percent of freestanding facilities have attained financial viability.

Freestanding facilities that provide ambulatory surgery procedures, commonly referred to as freestanding ambulatory surgery centers or surgicenters, have also proliferated. In 1987, it is estimated that 786 facilities performed approximately 1.5 million surgical procedures. In 1980, approximately 800 freestanding ambulatory surgery centers were operational; it is predicted that by 1990 approximately 1,200 such facilities will perform nearly 3 million surgical procedures.

Continued development of new technology and expanded payment policies for procedures performed in these settings will result in even more demand for facilities. Since 1982, the Health Care Financing Administration (HCFA) has increased the number of procedures reimbursed in facilities from 450 to more than 1,500. Many other players have followed HCFA's initiative, encouraging outpatient surgery in order to reduce costs of providing care and, in most cases, improve the quality of care as well. Similar to freestanding convenience clinics, ambulatory surgery centers have undergone much transformational change since their initial introduction. In many areas, centers have been developed in saturated markets for surgical caseloads, which has resulted in marginally profitable operations and consolidations with other facilities. Still, they represent a growing portion of a dynamic marketplace.

Finally, newer freestanding prototypes have been introduced for ambulatory programs and services, such as diagnostic imaging centers. These centers are the products of a combination of forces that have transformed traditional radiology from an inpatient service based on conventional X rays to a multimodal, technology-intensive service offered in a variety of settings. Currently, more than 20 percent of imaging procedures are now performed in freestanding settings, private radiology practices, and diagnostic imaging centers.

As technology continues to advance and payers increasingly seek more alternatives to control cost escalation, other types of freestanding facilities will emerge. This movement will no doubt continue despite the lack of empirical knowledge about whether these freestanding alternatives offer short-term savings or merely increase systemwide health care costs.

Office-Based Physician Practice

Solo and group office-based physician practice arrangements have long established themselves as the predominant deliverers of ambulatory care service. However, these entities are now experiencing the dramatic restructuring affecting other ambulatory care providers. Growth in the number of physicians is greater than population growth, physician practice affiliations are shifting as a result of increased competition, and cost-containment pressures are leading to more restrictive reimbursement policies. Currently, the practice of solo medicine is in decline, whereas physician group practices are experiencing phenomenal growth.

Group practices are emerging as increasingly powerful entities because larger patient volumes justify the acquisition of technologies once considered the domain of hospital-based ambulatory care programs. Generally, a group practice consists of three or more physicians who share the patient care and business aspects of a medical practice. The American Medical Association indicated that in 1987 physician group practices numbered 17,556, an increase of 61.3 percent since 1980.[3] Hospitals have shown an increasing interest in affiliating with or developing group practices in order to maintain and perhaps even increase market share. Hospitals have acknowledged widespread acquisition of group practices and entered into formalized joint venture relationships to ensure captivity of such markets.

The evidence of the powerful organization of group practices is apparent by the numerous large groups that have expanded to include not only traditional clinic-type operations, but also ambulatory surgery capabilities, diagnostic imaging services, urgent care programs, physical therapy, outpatient rehabilitation and sports medicine services, and cardiovascular diagnostic services. Because these groups are often the initial entrance point for a number of patients, they can offer ease and convenience for patients that hospitals and other freestanding providers are seeking to attract.

Historically, office-based practitioners have accounted for up to 40 percent of the total ambulatory care visits in the United States, including visits to hospitals and other freestanding ambulatory care facilities.[4] With the increasing movement toward multispecialty group practices, their survival will depend in part on their efforts to successfully deliver comprehensive, state-of-the-art services to ambulatory care patients.

In summary, the growth of ambulatory care supports strong evidence that the infrastructure of the health care industry is rapidly changing. Since implementation of the prospective payment system in 1983, hospitals have witnessed an ongoing erosion of inpatient admissions, declining lengths of stay, and revenues.

The Fragmentation of Ambulatory Care Services

The delivery system for ambulatory care services has become fragmented because recent changes in societal characteristics and values, expanding technology, and cost-containment initiatives have created multiple outpatient providers. Traditionally, the health care industry has been based upon the "cottage industry" model — the independent operations of physicians in private practice and hospitals as centers of delivery. This provider-controlled orientation led to systems being built primarily for inpatient care. Unfortunately, the traditional health care system can no longer support the sophisticated systems now required. Because many institutions have not yet begun positioning ambulatory care services for the future, their niche in the delivery system is no longer guaranteed. Hospitals have faced and will continue to face a period of major change. Ambulatory care will be an exceedingly challenging area in which to compete because it is now the preferred mode of patient care delivery, and there are low barriers to entry.

In the 1970s, hospitals enjoyed continued inpatient/outpatient growth and revenues. With the competitive era of the early 1980s, many hospitals witnessed the emergence of freestanding ambulatory care facilities. Often, these facilities were viewed with much skepticism by and received unfavorable attention from medical staff members. When these facilities posed competitive threats, hospitals responded by developing their own facilities or developing joint ventures with existing providers. Overall, hospitals were slow to adopt competitive postures and lost valuable market share; in some cases, this business was never regained.

Almost 20 years have passed since the first freestanding competitors emerged in hospital service areas. In 1990, some 45,000 freestanding ambulatory care settings are estimated to be operational, in contrast to nearly 8,000 providers in 1970, and nearly 6,000 hospitals that have traditionally provided the spectrum of ambulatory care services (table 1-2). This severe fragmentation of the marketplace is also dramatic in the number of patients treated per individual setting. Overall, the hospital ambulatory care marketplace has increased 98 percent during this 20-year period, from 181.4 million visits (1970) to 359.0 million visits (1990). These estimates do not reflect the number of office-based physician practices providing ambulatory and primary care, figures that would raise projections even higher.

Many health care policy experts have maintained that the current fragmentation of the ambulatory care industry is an indication that marketplace competition is successful. In some respects, this market philosophy is correct. Studies have shown that freestanding alternatives can offer similar services at lower costs than hospitals, because of lower overhead, lower administrative costs, and operational efficiency from a nonacute service orientation; that there is no evidence of quality-of-care differences between settings; and that patients sometimes prefer settings that are more conveniently located. Although some of these factors are measurable, there are significant aspects of ambulatory care service delivery about which very little is known yet but that have wide-ranging implications for national health policy and reimbursement. Of particular importance is the uncertainty about whether it is cost-effective to have multiple providers delivering services in numerous settings. In other words, as the fragmentation of providers and settings increases, what are the true effects on systemwide health care costs?

Table 1-2. Hospital-Based and Freestanding Ambulatory Care Providers, 1970–1990

	1970	1980	Estimated 1990
I. Hospital-based ambulatory care			
Total facilities	5,858	5,904	5,600
II. Freestanding ambulatory care			
Total providers	7,892	19,516	45,150
1. Freestanding ambulatory surgery centers	1	100	1,200
2. Freestanding ambulatory care centers	N/A	180	5,500
3. Diagnostic imaging centers	N/A	25	1,700
4. Industrial medicine clinics	N/A	5,000	8,000
5. Freestanding cancer centers	N/A	25	200
6. Mobile diagnostic units	N/A	50	750
7. Home care	N/A	2,924	5,800
8. Hospice	N/A	450	1,000
9. Physician group practice	7,891	10,762	21,000

Source: Division of Ambulatory Care and Health Promotion, American Hospital Association, 1989.

Critics argue that the total cost of care may be increased if the availability of freestanding facilities, in combination with existing hospital service capacity, causes either freestanding facilities or hospital programs and services to be underutilized. Thus, unnecessary duplication of service capacity and inefficient utilization of existing facilities could potentially add capital and operating costs to the total community cost of care.

Understanding the Cost Relationship

Because so little is known about the cost relationship between hospital-based and freestanding ambulatory care on the total community cost of care, it is clear that the fragmentation of ambulatory care that has only recently begun will no doubt continue for a significant period of time. Because fragmentation may eventually lead to severe restraints in the form of additional regulation, financial failure, and system consolidation, it is important to understand this cost relationship. Current developments and future implementation of ambulatory care services will largely depend on how this important issue is resolved.

None of the numerous quantitative research studies of hospital-based and freestanding ambulatory costs has been able to truly substantiate and differentiate costs of care in both settings. However, a critical examination of the study findings can best be described by using several hypotheses advanced by Altman and Socholitzky.[5] In their view, cost differences are thought to be a result of the following factors: (1) the accounting system used; (2) the facility's patient mix; and (3) economies of scale.

Accounting Systems

In considering the effect of accounting systems, it is important to remember that both hospital-based and freestanding ambulatory care settings are subject to cost reporting requirements of various agencies or institutions for purposes of reimbursement. As reported by Altman and Socholitzky, the problem of comparability of cost data stems from the differences in cost accounting systems used by hospital-based and freestanding ambulatory care facilities.

Because hospitals typically use costing methods that maximize reimbursement, the comparability of the cost data across different facilities is compromised. Freestanding facilities' costing practices differ widely from those used by hospitals. Because a freestanding ambulatory care facility is viewed as a single cost center, its costs will not be influenced by such things as the step-down approach or the allocation of overhead. These differences confound the problem inherent in comparing costs across different settings. Another problem in comparing the various research studies is that differences exist in the definitions of cost. For example, direct costs do not always refer to identical expense categories, and indirect costs may vary by site.

In 1979, Gold conducted an analysis of trends in the cost of care between hospital-based and freestanding ambulatory care facilities.[6] Despite data limitations and definitional ambiguities, Gold stated that there appears to be an implicit acceptance of the assumption that, based on figures current at the time, hospital-based primary care is generally more expensive than its freestanding counterpart. Many arguments have surfaced defending this position. Detmer stated, though not empirically, that the difference in costs between the two settings is one of technology.[7] Detmer suggested that freestanding ambulatory care facilities utilize less costly forms of technological intervention, thereby reducing the cost of care. In addition, ambulatory care in the hospital setting is different because it must share in the costs of high-tech inpatient care through the step-down accounting allocation process used by hospitals.

This argument leads to a second hypothesis, which states that the difference in costs is a result of the cost-accounting systems employed by many of the freestanding settings. Schultz identified three types of costs that may make hospital-based ambulatory care more expensive: (1) stand-by costs incurred by the hospital in providing certain services on a 24-hour or emergency basis; (2) by-product costs incurred because ambulatory care is included in the same financial system with more complex and extensive patient services; and (3) hidden costs incurred as a result of the cost allocation procedure and its concomitant inequitable distribution to ambulatory care.[8]

Facility–Patient Mix

In order to make a valid comparison of the costs of care across varied ambulatory settings, regardless of the method used to measure these costs, the characteristics of the patients being treated — the facility–patient mix — must be considered. The hypothesis frequently asserted is that hospital-based ambulatory care settings generally treat a sicker and demographically more complex patient than freestanding settings do. Gold stated that there are a number of reasons for thinking that the intensity of care provided in a hospital-based ambulatory care setting may be different, and possibly greater, than in the freestanding setting.[9] First, the hospital-based setting differs from the freestanding setting in that it may be viewed as an acute care facility whose major purpose has been to provide a more intensive level of care. This may affect a provider's orientation in delivering care, such as ordering more complex tests, additional consultations, and so forth. Second, as an extension of a hospital, the facility may also be viewed as an extension of the emergency department, drawing more severely ill patients and Medicare and Medicaid patients. Because these patients traditionally enter the health care delivery system at an extreme stage of illness, they will usually require a higher level of resources and, thereby, elevate costs.

Economies of Scale

In comparing the cost of ambulatory care across various facilities, it is clear that differences in cost may result from economies of scale. Epple and Reinhardt found that economies of scale existed in hospital-based settings and appeared to result from both lower input prices and an optimal mix of inputs.[10] The most relevant conclusion reached was that larger departments or facilities appear to have lower costs per patient and per visit, with the lowest costs achieved at 90,000 annual visits; clinics with fewer than 40,000 visits experienced severe cost disadvantages. Altman and Socholitzky stated that other factors compounding this issue include staffing patterns, actual productivity levels, underutilization of capacity, and stand-by costs.

In summary, a significant unresolved issue concerning the relationship between hospital-based and freestanding ambulatory care facilities is the true cost of services provided. Anecdotally, it appears that freestanding facilities are less expensive than their hospital-based counterparts, yet empirical results confirming this statement are nonexistent. In addition, the range and mix of procedures and the types of patients treated in both settings is unknown. The true cost of services provided is of critical importance for future policy and payment implications. The long-term impact of additional freestanding facilities may be an increase rather than a decrease in systemwide health care costs.

The lack of an understanding of cost differences means that hospital ambulatory care may quickly erode to multiple freestanding providers. In fact, under a fully prospective payment system, it can be argued that payers no longer consider cost of care an important distinction. Payment levels will be determined at fixed rates; profits will be derived only if providers fall within the payment threshold. Thus, hospitals must acknowledge that further splintering of ambulatory care sites will continue. To survive, hospitals will have to adopt competitive strategies similar to those that they have criticized their counterparts for embracing.

The Conflict between Inpatient and Outpatient Care

Traditionally, the health care delivery system in the United States has made inpatient care and services a higher priority than outpatient care and services. A great challenge lies ahead for hospitals to further develop and expand ambulatory care services that are both competitively structured and financially viable. In the past, because of the low priority given to ambulatory care services, the programs and services that were developed evolved not as a result of careful planning, but in response to immediate pressures from competitors or needs of medical staff members. As a result, hospital ambulatory care programs in the United States have been internally fragmented, causing overcrowding, inadequate access for patients, and operational inefficiency. In short, the reliance on developing systems primarily for inpatients has placed ambulatory care delivery at a great disadvantage. This conflict between inpatient and outpatient care must be resolved if hospitals are to successfully compete in the new health care environment.

The continuing fragmentation of ambulatory care delivery attests to the fact that hospitals have been improperly prepared to offer a competitive array of programs and services. For years, freestanding ambulatory care facilities have earned respect in the current delivery system by offering the mix of services demanded by consumers and others: convenience, multiple services offered in one location, competitive prices, ease of facility access, and an aesthetically pleasing environment.

Overall, inpatient care and outpatient care operate under different circumstances. This is important to understand, because different philosophies dictate separate courses of action. Forecasting ambulatory care utilization rates, for instance, is particularly difficult. Inpatient care has always operated under very structured requirements. Uniform statistical data reporting is required, which yields a multitude of state and national data sources, known use rates, historical trend reporting, and tracking. Conversely, ambulatory care utilization reporting is highly unstructured. Generally, uniform reporting is not a requirement; thus there are few state or national sources or established use rates available.

Finally, the operational characteristics of inpatient care and outpatient care vary widely. For hospitals, inpatient care has long been considered the core business and remains a primary focus, with ambulatory care as a distant second priority. In addition, hospitals use inpatient management to operate ambulatory care as well as existing inpatient systems for ambulatory operations. On the other hand, physicians continue to emphasize that ambulatory care is their primary domain of practice. Also, entrepreneurs approach ambulatory care as a primary market, emphasizing new managerial talent geared to ambulatory delivery as well as independent systems for ambulatory operations.

In light of the new realities of the marketplace, hospitals will have to reevaluate their primary mission, goals, and objectives. Although the hospital will always remain at the center of health care delivery, many institutions may redefine their primary mission, placing ambulatory care ahead of inpatient care. In any event, embarking on a strategy for reorganizing and integrating ambulatory care programs and services will require a long-term commitment to success.

Attributes of Successful Ambulatory Care Programs

The successful development or expansion of ambulatory care programs depends on many issues. Foremost among these, ambulatory care must be closely directed by an institution's top management, and there must be involvement of the board of trustees, medical staff members, and all departments providing ambulatory services. Yet this demonstration of commitment and involvement has largely been lacking until only recently.

Historically, the management structure and span of control of ambulatory care has varied by hospital bed size, complexity, academic affiliation, and geographic location, and has yet to be defined. In 1986, the Division of Ambulatory Care and Health Promotion of the American Hospital Association conducted a survey to quantify some of these relationships. The survey results indicated that ambulatory care programs were decentralized—51.1 percent of all ambulatory care programs offered were not under one management structure. Primary management control of ambulatory care resides principally with hospital administration (51.1 percent), followed by nursing administration (37.8 percent) and other managers (11.1 percent). Overall, 50 percent of ambulatory programs and facilities are managed by one administrator, but this is not the clear majority. Also, respondents indicated that the ambulatory care administrator may report directly to the hospital chief executive officer (40.8 percent); to the hospital chief operating officer (15 percent); to a hospital vice-president (13.1 percent); or to others (31.1 percent). This is an important distinction, as some contend that indirect reporting relationships to the hospital chief executive officer have hampered the development of ambulatory care activities.

Another important issue in the successful development and expansion of ambulatory care programs is organizational structure. In the late 1970s and early 1980s, corporate reorganizations were popular and provided hospitals with an opportunity to establish on a for-profit basis ambulatory care programs that had a separate tax status and governing authority from the hospital. Unfortunately, there has been surprisingly slow movement toward the reorganization of ambulatory care into a separate corporate structure. According to the American Hospital Association survey, corporate reorganization between 1975 and 1985 had occurred in only 26.8 percent of hospitals; 71 percent of these indicated that corporate reorganization did not involve ambulatory care programs. In addition, the majority of respondents, 71.7 percent, indicated there was no subsidiary entity that managed ambulatory diversification activities. For those indicating a subsidiary, the tax status of ventures was split between not-for-profit status (13.5 percent) and for-profit status (12.7 percent). From these results, it is clear that hospitals have not yet embraced the significance and importance of separating the organization, pricing, staffing, and operation of ambulatory care programs from those of acute care facilities. Many institutions are still of the opinion that the majority of revenue will be generated from the acute care service orientation.

Aside from top-level commitment and an appropriate organizational structure, successful ambulatory care also is dependent on several attributes that are unique to outpatient delivery. They include a readiness to compete aggressively in the marketplace, the development of programs and services that create adequate synergism to attract providers and patients, the correct mix of programs and services and the correct mix and number of professionals, and a strong commitment to provide outstanding service. These attributes apply generally to other forms of competitive health care delivery, but they are imperative for success in ambulatory care. This is because ambulatory care has two common problem areas that do not necessarily affect inpatient delivery: the location and the design of the facility. In terms of location, ambulatory care is often inconveniently located within or behind the hospital and difficult to gain access to; it is preferable that facilities be convenient, accessible, and highly visible. From a design point of view, ambulatory care facilities have not taken into account the growing number and mix of patients, which results in tremendous logistical and operational inefficiencies. Obviously, new systems must be designed to remedy these problem areas. The outcome, therefore, is the need to develop uncompromising facilities and services that focus on convenience, efficiency, cost competitiveness, attractiveness, continuity, productivity, high quality, and flexibility for both patients and providers.

Prototypes for the 1990s

Prototypes for the 1990s of successful ambulatory care programs must include a number of factors. As hospitals enter the next decade and compete for ambulatory care patients, there will be tremendous pressure to alter facility design arrangements in support of a consumer orientation. Specialized design for specific service areas, which can bring about high cost-effectiveness and operational efficiencies, as well as controlled overhead costs, is an issue at the cutting edge of ambulatory service development. It is becoming apparent that ambulatory facility design has an impact on direct cost of operation in relation to staffing, salaries, and fringe benefits, as well as on indirect overhead costs. It is becoming apparent that less viable options are to remodel or to use vacated space in the acute care institution to provide ambulatory services.

The responses of hospitals in this new era will be varied, dictated by such factors as geographic location, bed size, service offerings, and level of commitment. Some will have no other option than to renovate existing hospital space, whereas others will expand into additional freestanding environments or develop multidimensional facilities devoted exclusively to ambulatory care. Because of the recent fanfare about ambulatory care growth and the need to reorganize, a number of hospitals have adopted a competitive posture for ambulatory care. Increasingly, hospitals are making dramatic strides by restructuring and reorganizing all of their ambulatory care programs.

Examples of these efforts are illustrated by the rate of growth of new ambulatory care facilities. As shown in table 1-3, there were 281 ambulatory care facilities under development in 1988, an increase of 19.6 percent from 235 facilities in 1987. For diagnostic imaging centers, 230 facilities were planned or under construction in 1988, an increase of 40.2 percent from 164 in 1987. Finally, medical office buildings increased 16.9 percent, from 249 in 1987 to 291 in 1988.

Of the many and varied options available for ambulatory care expansion, the majority of facility developments in the future will no doubt be multidimensional in scope and design. Because ambulatory care is broad-based and highly complex in nature, service offerings will dictate the design of each facility. In addition, facilities increasingly will be developed on the campus of the main hospital. Rather than fragmented ambulatory care services, a multidimensional or integrated ambulatory care facility that centralizes ambulatory services in one location—the traditional hospital's health care campus—will no doubt be the preferred mode for service delivery.

The preference for a hospital campus and integrated ambulatory care facility is based on research of retail systems that have infrastructures that emphasize the clustering of products and services. This service option is attractive, convenient, efficient, and cost-competitive for both the customer and the provider. A full continuum of services is provided overall, and the various services still function independently and efficiently.

Obviously, the integrated ambulatory care facility is appearing in response to pressures and changes in the health care marketplace. It is important that upper-level management in health care organizations be flexible in responding to changes in delivery systems, especially in the area of ambulatory care.

Table 1-3.   Ambulatory Care Facility Development, 1987–1988

	1987	1988	Percentage Change
I. Ambulatory care center			
Completed	143	141	(1.4)
Under development	235	281	19.6
II. Diagnostic imaging center			
Completed	107	180	68.2
Under development	164	230	40.2
III. Medical office buildings			
Completed	152	155	23.7
Under development	249	291	16.9

Source: Adapted from *Modern Healthcare,* Construction and Architects Survey, 1989 and 1988.

References

1. American Hospital Association. *Outreach* 10(1), Jan.–Feb. 1989.
2. SMG Marketing Group, Inc. *Freestanding Ambulatory Care Center Report and Directory.* Chicago: SMG Marketing Group, Inc., June 1987.
3. American Medical Association. *Physician Characteristics and Distribution in the United States, 1987.* Chicago: AMA, 1987.
4. McLemore, T., and De Lozier, J. *1985 Summary: National Ambulatory Medical Care Survey. Advance Data.* Hyattsville, MD: National Center for Health Statistics, Jan. 23, 1987.
5. Altman, S., and Socholitzky, E. The cost of ambulatory care in alternative settings: a review of major research findings. *Annual Review of Public Health* 2:117–43, 1981.
6. Gold, M. Hospital-based versus freestanding primary care costs. *Journal of Ambulatory Care Management* 2:1–20, Feb. 1979.
7. Detmer, D. E. Ambulatory surgery. *New England Journal of Medicine* 305(23):2406–9, Dec. 1981.
8. Schultz, B. An analysis of hospital ambulatory care costs. Ph.D. dissertation, New York University, New York City, 1975.
9. Gold, pp. 1–20.
10. Epple, D., and Reinhardt, D. E. Analysis of the cost of ambulatory care at New York City hospitals. Unpublished report, Princeton University, Princeton, NJ, 1971.

Chapter 2

Rethinking Ambulatory Care Delivery

Theodore A. Matson

Overview of Ambulatory Care Services

The broad industry perspective of ambulatory care attests to the level of growth and expansion of specific programs and services. Each of these services is undergoing dramatic change and diversification. To understand its impact on individual hospitals and various providers, a separate analysis of each service offering is necessary. Only when providers recognize the impact of these areas can strategies be developed and implemented to ensure the competitive viability of all ambulatory care programs.

Ambulatory Surgery

Of all ambulatory services offered today, ambulatory surgery has experienced the greatest growth and has undergone the most profound changes. Preferred by an increasing number of third-party payers, physicians, and patients, ambulatory surgery eliminates the cost of a hospital stay and offers convenience to both physicians and patients.

The trend toward increased utilization of ambulatory surgery procedures persists for all hospital types, including not-for-profit and investor-owned hospitals. In 1987, 44 percent of procedures (9.8 million) were performed on an outpatient basis, an increase of 175 percent over 1980, when only 16 percent of procedures (3.2 million) were performed on an outpatient basis. Among hospital bed size groupings, all hospitals are now performing in excess of 40 percent outpatient procedures, with the exception of hospitals with more than 500 beds, which report 37 percent outpatient procedures. In various regions of the country, it has been reported that some hospitals are already reaching a 60 percent level of outpatient surgical procedures, which is predicted to be the industry average by 1995.[1] In terms of outpatient surgery by regions of the country, all hospitals again are performing in excess of 40 percent of surgical procedures on an outpatient basis. As shown in table 2-1, the proportion of outpatient procedures ranges from 40 percent in the East South Central region to 49 percent in the New England region. These figures are quite dramatic, considering that as recently as 1984 only the New England, East North Central, and Mountain regions posted outpatient surgical percentages greater than 30 percent.

The proliferation of freestanding surgical centers, estimated to number approximately 786 in 1987, has caused an obvious erosion of some patients from traditional hospital-based programs. Although freestanding surgical centers performed 1.5 million procedures in 1987, hospitals still hold approximately an 85 to 90 percent share of the surgical procedure market.[2]

This trend is important, as freestanding facilities now operate in a matured marketplace following moderate expansion since the 1970s.

Continued development of new technologies and expanded payment initiatives for ambulatory surgery, including increased provider (physician) acceptance, will no doubt shift the majority of previous inpatient caseloads to outpatient settings. The number of surgical procedures that can be appropriately conducted in outpatient environments, often a subject of great debate, now exceeds one thousand in number. As shown in figure 2-1, the list of common procedures that can be performed on an outpatient basis is wide-ranging. According to a 1987 survey conducted by the American Hospital Association's Division of Ambulatory Care and Health Promotion, the most commonly performed procedures are cataract procedures with lens insertion (11.7 percent), dilation and curettage (10.5 percent), erosion of skin lesion (9.1 percent), arthroscopy (6.4 percent), tubal ligation (5.4 percent), laparoscopy (4.9 percent), myringotomy (4.8 percent), and tonsillectomy (3.9 percent), with other procedures comprising the remaining number (43.7 percent).

Table 2-1. Percentage of Surgery Done on an Ambulatory Basis by Region, 1987

West North Central	46.0
West South Central	41.0
East North Central	48.0
East South Central	40.0
New England	49.0
Middle Atlantic	42.0
South Atlantic	44.0
Pacific	43.0

Source: *Annual Survey of Hospitals, American Hospital Association, 1987.* Chicago: American Hospital Association, 1987.

Figure 2-1. Surgical Procedures That Can Be Performed on an Outpatient Basis

Dental
Multiple teeth extraction, first hour
    each additional hour
Periodontal surgery, first hour

Ear, Nose, Throat
A and M windows
Adenoidectomy
Adenoidectomy w/myringotomy (U)
Adenoidectomy w/myringotomy (B)
Arch bars, removal
Brachial arch appendages, excision
    (brachial cyst)
Bronchoscopy
Bronchoscopy w/biopsy
Caldwell-Luc
Ear examination
Esophagoscopy
Esophagoscopy w/biopsy
Ethmoidectomy
Foreign body removal from ear
Inclusion cyst, excision
Inferior turbinate resection
Jaw, closed reduction and fixation
Laryngoscopy
Laryngoscopy w/biopsy
Mouth biopsy
Myringoplasty or tympanoplasty
Myringotomy w/T&A (B)
Myringotomy w/wo tubes (U)
Myringotomy w/wo tubes (B)
Nasal bones, open reduction
Nasal bones, closed reduction
Nasal polypectomy
Otoscopy
Otoscopy w/foreign body removal
Palate biopsy
Poly tubes removal
Preauricular cyst excision
Septal reconstruction, SMR
Tonsillar tag excision
Tonsillectomy w/wo adenoidectomy
Tongue biopsy
Wedge resection, lip
Zygoma/zygomatic arch, open reduction

Eyes
Cataract extraction
Cataract extraction with lens insertion

Chalazion excision
Conjunctiva, lesion excision repair
Dermoid cyst, eyebrow excision
Ectropion or entropion repair
Enucleation of eye
Examination, eye (tray charge)
Eyelid lesion excision
Lacrimal duct excision
Lacrimal duct probing
Lacrimal duct reconstruction
Laser treatment
Muscle surgery, eye (U)
Muscle surgery, eye (B)
Pterygium (U)
Pterygium (B)
Resection, recession (U)
Resection, recession (B)

General Surgery
Abscess I&D
Baker's cyst excision (behind knee)
Breast mass, excision biopsy (U)
Breast mass, excision biopsy (B)
Cervical node biopsy
Colostomy revision
Cyst excision, simple or 1
Cyst excision, multiple or complex
Dermoid cyst excision
Epigastric herniorrhaphy
Fistulectomy
Fissurectomy
Foreign body removal w/o x-ray
Foreign body removal w/x-ray
Frenulectomy, tongue
Gastroscopy
Gastrostomy revision or closure
Granuloma
Gynecomastia, excision (U)
Gynecomastia, excision (B)
Hemangioma removal
Hematoma
Hemorrhoidectomy
Hernia repair, incisional
Herniorrhaphy, inguinal (U)
    Infant (up to 2 years)
    Adult (2 years and older)
Herniorrhaphy, femoral (U)
Herniorrhaphy, femoral (B)

Continued on next page

Figure 2-1. (Continued)

Laceration repair, under 1 hour
Laceration repair, over 1 hour
Lipoma & mass (lesion, nodule) excision
Lymph node biopsy
Lesion, multiple excision, over 1 hour
Lesion, excision, under 1 hour
Melanoma excision
Mole excision (tray charge)
Muscle biopsy
Orchiectomy
Pilonidal cyst excision
Rectal biopsy
Rectal dilation (tray charge)
Rectal polypectomy
Rectal fistula repair
Sigmoidoscopy (tray charge)
Sigmoidoscopy w/biopsy and/or anesthesia
Skin grafting, simple
Skin grafting, complex
Suture removal, superficial (tray charge)
Suture removal, deep
Thyroglossal duct cyst excision
Umbilical herniorrhaphy
Umbilical herniorrhaphy w/inguinal
 repair (U)
Umbilical herniorrhaphy
Umbilical herniorrhaphy repair (B)
Varicose vein ligation
Varicose vein ligation w/stripping (U)
Varicose vein ligation w/stripping (B)
Vermilionectomy
Wedge lip resection

Gynecology
Bartholin cyst, excision
Cervical biopsy
Cervical cerclage
Cervical conization
Cervical dilatation
Cervical polyp excision
Clitoris lysis or adhesions
Colpotomy (vaginal tubal ligation)
Condyloma accuminata excision
Cryotherapy, cervix (tray charge)
Cryotherapy, w/biopsy or D&C
Culdocentesis
Culdoscopy
Dilatation and curettage (D&C)
 D&C, cauterization cervix
 D&C, w/cone

 D&C, w/hysteroscopy
Eder Hasson
Embryo transfer
Fulguration of condyloma accuminata
Hymenotomy
Hymen reconstruction
Hysteroscopy
IUD removal (tray charge)
Labia, excision lesions
Laparoscopy, diagnostic
Laparoscopy, follicular aspiration
Laparoscopy, open, w/Hasson Eder
Laparoscopy w/aspiration fluid
Laparoscopy w/biopsy
Laparoscopy w/D&C or tubal
Laparoscopy w/dye studies
Laparoscopy w/lysis of adhesions
Laparotomy w/tubal sterilization (B)
Laparotomy, mini
Pelvic examination, under anesthesia
Perineoplasty
Perineorrhaphy
Transvaginal tubal ligation
Vaginal septum, incision and/or excision
Vaginal tumor excision
Vaginoplasty
Vaginoscopy
Vulva lesion, excision/biopsy
Vulvectomy, partial
Urethral carbuncle
Laparoscopy, follicular aspiration
Embryo transfer

Neurosurgery
Carpal tunnel decompression
Morton's neuroma excision
Neurolysis, ulnar, elbow, w/wo transfer
Neuroma (other) excision

Orthopedics
Amputation or revision, finger
Amputation or revision, toe
Arthrodesis, finger
Arthrodesis, toe
Arthrotomy w/joint exploration
Arthrotomy w/meniscectomy
Arthroscopy, knee
 Diagnostic
 Ligament repair
 Meniscectomy
 Synovectomy

Figure 2-1. (Continued)

Bone graft
Bone reconstruction
Bunionectomy (U)
Bunionectomy (B)
Bunionectomy w/implant
Bursectomy, olecranon
Bursectomy, patellar

Plastic Surgery
Augmentation mammoplasty (U)
Augmentation mammoplasty (B)
Blepharoplasty, upper or lower (B)
Blepharoplasty, combined or quad
Chemical peel, full face
Chemical peel, lips
Chin augmentation
Dermabrasion, full face
Dermabrasion, partial
Lipectomy, abdominal (local)
Lipectomy, abdominal (general)
Lipectomy, submental
Mastoplexy, simple

Mastoplexy, complex (U)
Mastoplexy, complex (B)
Mini face-lift
Otoplasty (U)
Otoplasty (B)
Rhinoplasty
Rhinoplasty tip
Rhytidectomy (face-lift)
Rhytidectomy w/blepharoplasty
Vermilionectomy, upper or lower lip
Vermilionectomy, combined
Xanthoma, upper or lower lid (B)
Xanthoma, combined
Suction-assisted lipectomy:
  Abdomen
  Arm
  Buttocks
  Hip
  Thighs
  Chin

U = unilateral
B = bilateral

Technological enhancements notwithstanding, perhaps the greatest movement toward outpatient surgery for hospitals will result from the enactment of the Federal Omnibus Reconciliation Act of 1986. This measure calls for the development of a prospective payment system (PPS) for reimbursing all Medicare outpatient services, and until fully implemented, sets forth new regulations for reimbursing hospitals for providing ambulatory surgical services to Medicare beneficiaries. Section 943(a) of the Omnibus Budget Reconciliation Act (OBRA) requires that, for cost reporting periods beginning on or after October 1, 1987, Medicare payment for certain ambulatory surgical procedures performed in a hospital on an outpatient basis be based in part on what the government would have paid for the same procedure if it had been performed in an approved ambulatory surgical center (ASC). Reimbursement will be based on a combination of the ASC rate and a blending of each hospital's reasonable cost and customary charges.

Several key features of these regulations will force hospitals to implement operational changes to accommodate the medical records, billing, information systems, and other requirements to ensure payment. One important characteristic of the new payment methodology is the actual definition of what constitutes an ambulatory surgical procedure.

Surgery is defined by the Health Care Financing Administration (HCFA) as any incision, excision, amputation, introduction, repair, destruction, suture, or manipulation. This includes some procedures, such as endoscopic examinations, that hospitals might not consider within the domain of true ambulatory surgical procedures. Under the broad definition imposed by HCFA, surgical procedures can occur in a multitude of settings, such as the emergency department, outpatient clinics, and in departments where such interventional procedures as radiology are performed. Hospitals should identify each of these areas, capture costs on a per-visit basis, and develop methods to identify the mix of these patients in terms of the adopted case-mix classification scheme.

A second important feature of OBRA is that outpatient procedures must be coded according to HCFA's Common Procedural Coding System (HCPCS). Each procedure must be coded, whether or not it is an ASC-approved procedure. Hospitals will be required to continue submitting ICD-9-CM diagnosis codes; however, ICD-9 procedural codes are no longer required. The Health Care Financing Administration has stated that it will use an Outpatient Code Editor that will edit the UB-82 form and will reject those claims that are miscoded. To this end, providers will have to develop management information systems that provide a "crosswalk" between coding systems, as well as conversion tables to expedite the interface between coding systems.

Although the current Medicare payment mechanisms for surgery-related services have been cited by HCFA as having several shortcomings, a fully prospective system for reimbursing outpatient surgery is mandated to be implemented by OBRA. According to an interim report in 1988, HCFA officials have indicated that the same basic methodology should be used to develop a prospective payment system of rates for similar surgical procedures, regardless of whether the procedure is performed in a hospital outpatient setting or in a freestanding facility. In addition, the design of a new system would need to incorporate: (1) the selection of a surgical procedure or episode of care that corresponds with the services utilized; and (2) an adjusting mechanism to the Medicare payment price to account for cost differences among providers and suppliers of these services.

Regardless of the specific methodology chosen by HCFA, the U.S. government recognizes the need to create incentives for efficiency and productivity. Currently, Medicare charges for outpatient surgery are approximately 20 percent of total outpatient charges. The continued growth in utilization and the resulting expenditures will force the nation's hospitals to rethink the delivery of these services and improve the financial viability of their programs.

Emergency Department Services

Emergency departments provide a mix of services for both emergency patients and patients requiring primary medical care. Among all settings, emergency departments have become the location of choice of patients seeking care for urgent medical conditions and minor episodic injuries. The amount and type of primary care services provided by emergency departments are greatly influenced by whether or not an individual hospital operates an organized outpatient department or other ambulatory care programs and by the organizational characteristics and range of services provided.

Despite the emergency department's role in providing care to great numbers of outpatients, many institutions consider the emergency department to be an inpatient service. This is because the emergency department is the single largest source of inpatient admissions. Currently, 30 percent of total hospital admissions nationwide are generated by the emergency department. Similarly, 10 to 20 percent of emergency department visits result in an inpatient admission. In addition to representing nearly 30 percent of total ambulatory care utilization in hospitals, emergency departments also account for significant volumes of other diagnostic/ancillary utilization. It is estimated that as much as 60 percent of outpatient radiology procedures and as much as 40 percent of outpatient laboratory procedures are generated by emergency department patients.[3]

During the past several years, hospital emergency departments have witnessed erosion in visits of some patients. Most dramatically, from 1981 to 1984, emergency department utilization nationwide decreased by approximately 10 percent on average; some hospitals witnessed declines of as much as 30 percent.[4] In 1986, the American Hospital Association's Division of Ambulatory Care and Health Promotion conducted a survey of reasons for declining emergency department utilization as well as operational measures implemented to correct declining visits. When asked to determine what factors contributed to a decline in patients, those polled indicated the following: competition from freestanding convenience clinics (30 percent), expanded physician office hours (25 percent), health maintenance organization (HMO) and preferred provider organization (PPO) plans that discourage emergency department use (20 percent), competing emergency departments (10 percent), reimbursement patterns of insurers (10 percent), and the reduction of in-house primary care services (5 percent).

In response to these threats, nearly 50 percent of emergency departments reported that they have either completed or were planning to implement a restructuring of patient charges (tiered pricing) in order to meet the competition. Nearly the same percentage indicated they had either implemented or were planning to develop a separate program or area to expedite treatment of nonurgent patients. Often referred to as "fast-track" programs, this concept is viewed as an alternative to freestanding facilities. These centers offer lower cost and walk-in services, with the added marketing advantage of being open 24 hours a day and having the full back-up capabilities of comprehensive services if required.

Since the implementation of these competitive strategies and techniques, hospitals have witnessed moderate to strong growth in recapturing patients previously lost to alternative providers. In some instances, dramatic growth has occurred and hospitals are experiencing the highest level of utilization ever recorded. And in some highly competitive markets, hospitals have forced freestanding convenience clinics to close or to consolidate with other providers. For others, the combination of increased utilization and more equitable product-costing of services has yielded a return to departmental profitability.

Despite the success that emergency departments now enjoy, the future will bring many challenges. Today, there is growing concern among many third-party payers that emergency departments are inappropriately utilized, causing unneeded and costly expenditures. Critics contend that as many as 70 percent of current emergency department patients could be treated in more appropriate, cost-effective settings. Various payers are now implementing more stringent requirements as to what constitutes an appropriate versus an inappropriate patient visit, and increasingly are denying payment for certain types of services. In addition, a number of HMO and PPO plans now discourage emergency department use and have begun to institute deductibles for patients who are inappropriately referred for emergency department care.

As these cost-containment strategies become widespread, national emergency department utilization will stabilize and then begin to decline. It is projected by the American Hospital Association that emergency department visits will stabilize by 1990 and then decrease for several years.[5] This trend will in turn have a negative financial impact on hospitals. The American Hospital Association estimates that emergency departments contribute 3 to 7 percent of hospital revenues directly and contribute as much as 45 percent of revenues indirectly through ancillaries, patient days, and supplies.[6] To survive in this environment, hospitals will have to ensure that their emergency departments are oriented toward the consumer; pricing of services must be based on the actual cost of providing such care, and some services that do not achieve profitability may have to be eliminated or merged with other facilities.

Diagnostic Radiology and Imaging

Radiologic diagnostic and imaging capabilities have emerged as one of the most exciting and challenging areas in hospital outpatient expansion during the past five years. Diagnostic radiology imaging has been transformed from a level of routine, diagnostic technology to one that is based on a high-technology approach. The shift of traditional diagnostic examinations to such digital modalities as magnetic resonance imaging (MRI), computerized tomography (CT), and ultrasound will forever change the landscape of radiological technology. Future advances in development of multimodal techniques will greatly affect the treatment regimens of patients and move diagnostic radiology/imaging into the forefront as one of the first tools to be incorporated in the diagnosis and management of patients. The emergence of positron emission tomography (PET) imaging, which provides three-dimensional metabolic and functional views of organs, and lithotripsy, which uses "shock wave" ultrasound to destroy kidney stones and gallstones, are but two examples.

The provision of radiology and diagnostic imaging services is challenged by the manner in which these services can be provided. In addition to hospital-based radiology departments, services increasingly are being developed in freestanding imaging centers and on the road via mobile vans. For hospitals, this is a difficult situation, for radiology departments often suffer financial losses because of the high overhead associated with their staffing and technology costs. As lower-cost, high-volume procedures are provided outside the hospital, higher costs per in-hospital procedure are incurred, which increases the level of operating losses.

Although technology will bring additional radiology patients and revenues, reimbursement for these services will be reduced in the future. In particular, the Federated Omnibus Reconciliation Act of 1987 will place reimbursement limits on outpatient diagnostic and therapeutic radiology services. Effective for all cost reporting periods beginning on or after October 1, 1987, Medicare payments for hospital outpatient radiology services are limited to the lesser of the hospital's reasonable costs or customary charges, or a blended amount of reasonable costs and a portion of the prevailing charges paid to participating physicians who perform the service in their offices in the same locality. Radiology services that are included under these provisions include diagnostic and therapeutic radiology, CT, MRI, nuclear medicine, ultrasound, and other imaging services.

Since October 1, 1989, the prevailing charge has been based on a relative value scale (RVS) set by the Health Care Financing Administration. Thus, Medicare will determine what is usual, reasonable, and customary based on a fee schedule that reflects averaged regional fees. This new rate structure has several important characteristics. First, the cost proportion is defined as the actual reasonable cost, from a technical standpoint, to perform a radiology service. The cost proportion will account for 65 percent of the total amount billed to Medicare in fiscal year 1989. The amount will be reduced to 50 percent in subsequent years. Second, the charge proportion of the formula, the physician's professional charge, will represent 35 percent of billing in fiscal year 1989 and 50 percent thereafter. Third, the charge proportion of the entire bill will be 62 percent of 80 percent of the prevailing charges for physicians performing identical services in the same geographic region. In other words, HCFA has assumed that 62 percent of the cost of radiology services performed in a physician's office represents all the costs of providing a radiologic service other than the fee charged by the physician.

Overall, this interpretation means that the technical component of the reimbursable charge will be less for hospitals than under the current system because of the higher overhead rate that is characteristic of outpatient radiology departments. Generally, the RVS rates are expected to have a larger impact on those hospitals that perform general diagnostic procedures; specialized imaging services, such as CT and ultrasound, will be less affected. Thus, hospitals that operate diversified imaging programs will fare better than single-modality programs.

In the future, hospitals must brace themselves for the pending reimbursement challenges. Strategies employed to assist in operational decision making should include cost accounting of services to more precisely define departmental productivity; profit-and-loss analyses for each imaging modality to determine whether certain cost controls should be employed; and consideration of new alternatives to acquire technology or increase departmental profitability, such as equipment leasing, contract management, and joint ventures. Local and regionalized service offerings, such as multi-institutional development of MRI services, may be the only alternative for some institutions to achieve profitable operations.

Clinical Laboratory Testing

Clinical laboratory testing, provided in hospitals, physicians' offices, and independent laboratories, is one aspect of ambulatory care services that is undergoing rapid change on a daily basis. It is a fiercely competitive marketplace, with seemingly endless numbers of providers in a matured environment.

Even though clinical laboratory testing is an enormous industry, the exact number of tests performed by the various testing entities is unknown. It is estimated, however, that the market is approximately $20 billion annually, with the biggest share — $13 million — provided by hospitals.[7] Approximately 6 billion tests are performed annually; 50 to 57 percent of tests are performed in hospitals, 25 to 30 percent are performed in independent laboratories, and the remaining 15 to 20 percent are conducted in physicians' offices. According to the most recent estimates, 74 percent of all clinical laboratories in the United States have witnessed increasing volumes in tests conducted since 1984–1986. In the future, it is predicted that hospital laboratory testing will increase at an annual rate of 5 percent, whereas laboratory testing in physicians' offices and group practices will experience annual growth of 16 and 19 percent, respectively.

Historically, total laboratory testing over the past three decades has consistently achieved double-digit figures. Although growth will continue in the future, massive restructuring and consolidation among the various players will proliferate. For hospitals, ongoing changes in payment systems are transforming laboratories from profit centers to cost centers. Prior to the implementation of the prospective payment system, hospital laboratories generated approximately 12 percent of total hospital revenue; laboratories now cost money instead of generating it.[8]

Overall, the number of hospital and independent laboratories has decreased more than 30 percent in the past decade as a result of consolidations, acquisitions, and joint ventures between competitors. These changes are primarily due to the fact that profits are directly related to economies of scale; most tests provide slim profit margins and are dependent on tremendous volume to ensure financial viability. Conversely, the number of physician office laboratories has increased dramatically, as has the range of testing available in these offices. This growth has occurred because of patients' and physicians' desires for quicker turnaround of tests, enhanced medical technology that has made office testing easier, and a somewhat favorable reimbursement climate that has helped boost the profitability of such laboratories.[9]

In the future, cost pressures and reimbursement challenges will continue to threaten the operational effectiveness of hospital laboratory testing. More tests will be provided on a decentralized basis because of the development of simple instrumentation and test kits that allow tests to be performed by patients at home. To remain active players in the field, hospitals will have to implement a number of innovative strategies. First, productivity and efficiency will be the keys to cost reduction. Viable options to consider include the use of independent laboratories for certain types of testing, contract management to assume the costs of laboratory training programs, equipment upgrading, computerization of testing and results reporting, and overall administration of the laboratory department. In addition, a structure may be created that enables the hospital to act as a reference laboratory for physicians and industry.

In what is perhaps a more far-reaching strategy, hospitals may relentlessly delegate certain types of testing to their formally or informally organized medical staff members who operate satellite facilities. Although this strategy will lead to an erosion of market share and income, the movement of testing to outside the hospital is inevitable; a joint venture structure under which profits are shared is thus an acceptable strategy. Further support for a joint venture strategy will materialize because physician offices will no doubt rely on hospital laboratories to a certain extent, as new legislation will require physician laboratories to meet various proficiency and quality standards.

Cardiovascular Services

Cardiovascular services are perhaps the largest market segment in health care, because heart disease is the number one cause of death in the United

States, and more than 65 million individuals have cardiovascular disease. Yet, the growth of this market is only just beginning; the role of ambulatory care as a delivery site for cardiovascular services largely remains untapped.

Historically, cardiology services in hospitals have focused primarily on such inpatient services as cardiac catheterization and cardiovascular surgery. Today, although these invasive procedures have served as the cornerstone of cardiovascular services, noninvasive procedures performed on an ambulatory care basis are leading current program development and expansion efforts. Furthermore, some invasive procedures that were once considered to be only the domain of inpatient services, such as cardiac catheterization, are being performed in limited numbers in the ambulatory setting. In short, as technology and provider acceptance increase, ambulatory care will be looked upon as an appropriate alternative to providing cardiovascular services in dedicated inpatient settings. Outpatient departments and freestanding settings will also benefit from payer concerns and directives that services should be performed in the most appropriate and cost-effective environments.

Currently, outpatient cardiovascular services consist of many diagnostic modalities, including electrocardiography (ECG), stress electrocardiography, echocardiography, nuclear cardiology, and noninvasive vascular imaging. Over the past decade, noninvasive cardiology services have been growing rapidly. The additions of echocardiography and nuclear cardiography have been the leading reasons for this growth. Recently, the addition of noninvasive vascular imaging has increased awareness of the extent to which new technology can generate much-needed revenues from diagnosing vascular-related disorders.

In addition to the expansion of outpatient cardiovascular testing services, growth in the next ten years will come from the relocation of inpatient services to the outpatient setting. Diagnostic cardiac catheterization, discussed previously, is the best example of this shift in service provision. Because the majority of hospitals with comprehensive cardiology services have yet to endorse cardiac catheterization on an outpatient basis, freestanding cardiac catheterization facilities provide these services almost exclusively.

Independent cardiac catheterization facilities are less common than their freestanding counterparts, such as freestanding imaging centers. In fact, some states have strict prohibitions against these facilities, whereas in other regions of the country there are few operating restrictions. Generally, in states where they are allowed, freestanding catheterization facilities are treated the same as any other roentgenographic facility or service that is performed in a physician's office. In other states, pilot projects funded under legislative sponsorship are under way. In each instance, the goal of such efforts is to determine whether these facilities are cost-effective alternatives to more expensive inpatient settings.

Outpatient cardiac catheterization has also been developed via mobile laboratories; however, use of these mobile units has been limited to situations in which existing laboratories are being refurbished or new facilities are under construction. The technology is essentially the same as that found in mobile CT and MRI services and is used in areas where a full-time, dedicated catheterization laboratory is not yet warranted. In the future, it is reasonable to expect that some areas, especially rural ones, may be well served by this technology. Once this complex procedure gains acceptance by more providers and institutions, other cardiovascular procedures will see the outpatient setting become the setting of choice.

Comprehensive Cancer Care

Industry estimates indicate that cancer accounts for 10 percent of the total cost of disease in the United States, and that 30 percent of the population will develop some form of cancer.[10] Because of the increasing incidence of cancer over time and the effects of today's competitive arena, many hospitals have become interested in establishing formally organized centers for the diagnosis and treatment of cancer disorders.

In 1988, the Division of Ambulatory Care and Health Promotion of the American Hospital Association conducted an industry survey to determine the extent of hospital involvement in providing oncology services. According to the survey, 32 percent of hospitals in the United States provide outpatient cancer care services. Hospitals with between 100 and 300 beds reported the greatest degree of involvement in these services (32 percent); 23 percent of hospitals with fewer than 100 beds indicated involvement in cancer programs. In addition, 60 percent of hospital cancer care programs were developed after 1981. This clearly indicates the extent to which hospital executives responded to environmental forces by providing cancer care services.

In terms of patient utilization, the typical hospital outpatient cancer program services approximately 160 newly diagnosed outpatients per month and provides 1,200 direct outpatient visits, or 7.0 visits per patient per month. Radiation therapy accounted for 55 percent of total visits, assessments and consultations for 10 percent, physical therapy for 7 percent, surgery for 6 percent, social services for 5 percent, occupational therapy for 4 percent, patient education for 3 percent, and speech therapy for 2 percent of total visits. In addition, 53 percent of cancer patients are female, and 51 percent are under 65 years of age. The top six diagnostic categories treated in hospital cancer programs are lung, breast, colorectal, gynecological, prostate, and leukemia and lymphomas. Patients with acquired immunodeficiency syndrome (AIDS) were treated in 53 percent of hospital cancer programs.

Unfortunately, the survey results reflect a delivery system for outpatient cancer care that is seriously fragmented, provided in a multitude of settings, managed by numerous individuals, and generally provided in an uncoordinated fashion. This contrasts with the perceived benefit of a comprehensive cancer care program — one that is multidisciplinary in treatment protocols and personnel and includes full radiation therapy capabilities, support services, a tumor registry, and outpatient chemotherapy services.

In the future, for hospitals to remain competitive in the market for outpatient cancer care, they must adopt the strategies that their competitors — for example, freestanding cancer centers and private oncologists' offices — have incorporated. This includes a dedicated area or building that centralizes all multidisciplinary activities, is consumer-oriented in appearance and designed for efficient patient flow, and is aesthetically pleasing to patients.

Emphasis must also be placed on ensuring the operational efficiency of the outpatient cancer care program in order to sustain financial viability. Medicare is the single largest payer of hospital outpatient cancer care services, accounting for 43 percent of a typical program's total revenue. In 1987, the Health Care Financing Administration began reforming policies concerning the reimbursement of outpatient cancer centers. The Health Care Financing Administration modified a long-standing policy that allowed physicians to be paid for daily management services for radiation oncology patients, even when the physicians did not treat the patients personally. Under the new directive, physicians in an outpatient cancer center must actually see patients in order to be reimbursed.

Other changes in Medicare outpatient reimbursement affect the level of profitability of outpatient cancer care services as well. Since October 1, 1988, outpatient radiology services have been reimbursed at a rate calculated by blending hospital-specific costs and physician charges. In the first year, the blend consisted of 65 percent hospital-specific costs and 35 percent based on 62 percent of the amount physicians received. Starting October 1, 1989, the blend was adjusted to 50 percent of hospital-specific costs and 50 percent of physician charges. Finally, the creation of a fully prospective payment system for outpatient services by 1991, including a case-mix classification schema for outpatient cancer services, will further erode reimbursement from some programs and providers.

Medical Rehabilitation

Medical rehabilitation has become increasingly important in the past few years because of recognition of its potential in patient care and cost pressures from payers as a result of the prospective payment system. During this period, there has been growth in all entities that provide rehabilitation services. These include inpatient rehabilitation beds, rehabilitation hospitals, skilled nursing facilities, comprehensive outpatient rehabilitation facilities (CORFs), home care agencies that provide rehabilitation services, and rehabilitation agencies.

Generally, medical rehabilitative care involves clinical, functional, social, and welfare assessment, followed by a coordinated approach to the patient's total management. It is multidisciplinary in nature, in that many allied health personnel are involved in each patient's care plan. A number of professionals are involved, including physicians, physiatrists, physical therapists, occupational therapists, social workers, psychologists, orthotists, speech therapists, nurses, and vocational counselors. Because of its complex structure, medical rehabilitation has been a segment of the health care industry that has been poorly understood. Now, however, insurers and other payers are taking a more positive view of rehabilitation. In addition, hospitals now realize the profit opportunities that these services can offer.

In the future, because of the aging of the population, advancing medical techniques, and increased survival of severely injured or ill persons (such as those with head injury trauma and congenitally disabled patients), medical rehabilitation will expand greatly. However, with patient expansion in these programs, rising expenditures will be closely monitored and alternatives to reducing costs of care for rehabilitation patients will be pursued. Of the many facilities that are available to rehabilitation patients, comprehensive outpatient rehabilitation facilities (CORFs) will emerge as primary deliverers of rehabilitation care.

Comprehensive outpatient rehabilitation facilities may provide care to multiple types of rehabilitative patients, or they may specialize in management of specific cases, such as cardiac rehabilitation, head injury rehabilitation, pediatric rehabilitation, worker rehabilitation, and industrial rehabilitation. The specialization approach is significant, because a regionalized program devoted to a specific patient mix can yield large volumes of patients. For example, head injury cases constitute one of the most interesting niches in rehabilitation. According to the National Head Injury Foundation, only 26 percent of the 70,000 to 90,000 patients with severe head injuries get specialized treatment each year.[11] In addition, 500,000 individuals who sustain minor head injuries each year and need to be monitored and treated in sophisticated treatment centers do not have access to these centers because of their lack of availability.

With the potential development of a prospective payment system for treating rehabilitation patients, it is conceivable that only acutely ill patients will remain in hospital rehabilitation centers. The remaining patients will be treated in the various other settings available, with hospital outpatient programs treating the majority of patients. Hospitals must take the initiative in developing and expanding these specialized services in the future because rehabilitative patients will comprise a significant percentage of all ambulatory patients. Competition for these patients will be extremely fierce; some providers will be able to deliver care comparable to hospital care at lower costs.

Specialty Outpatient Clinics

Environmental forces, changing technology, and declining reimbursement have greatly encouraged ambulatory care growth. Recent diversification into new forms of outpatient delivery options, such as occupational health, industrial medicine, and women's health services, have continued expansion efforts. In the future, additional forms of ambulatory care services will be delivered as a result of specialization in various disorders and various diseases. Examples include allergies and asthma, arthritis, diabetes, digestive diseases, pain management resulting from diseases, and sleep disorders.

Allergy Disorders

Approximately 14 percent of the population, 35 million individuals, suffer from allergy- and asthma-related disorders.[12] The interest in these programs has blossomed because of growing awareness of the severity and increased incidence of these conditions in the past ten years. For instance, asthma deaths in children have doubled during this period; treating asthma also is becoming more complicated because of the number of new medications on the market. Generally, allergy programs require a physician specialist in allergies and asthma treatment; however, minimal equipment is required for the programs.

Arthritis

Approximately 45 million Americans suffer from some form of arthritis.[13] As the population ages, the diagnosis and treatment of arthritis conditions will be in even greater demand. Generally, a formally organized arthritis treatment program consists of a team of professionals, including a rheumatologist who is a specialist in arthritis disorders, an orthopedist, an occupational therapist, a physical therapist, a pharmacist, a dietitian, and an exercise physiologist. Services offered consist of comprehensive screening to determine the presence and extent of arthritis; therapeutic intervention; health maintenance outpatient services, such as physical and occupational therapy; and educational services. Hospitals often will find that their programs are well received by patients because they can receive all services in one setting.

Diabetes

Diabetes also is a major health problem in the United States, affecting approximately 11 million Americans of whom approximately 6 million are unaware that they have the disease.[14] Of the current diabetes treatment programs in hospitals, the vast majority have focused on the provision of care to inpatients. Because of the enormous numbers of individuals who as yet have not been diagnosed with the disease, future programs will strongly emphasize ambulatory care testing as well as management of patients on an ambulatory basis. Diabetes treatment programs are similar in organization and scope of services offered to other specialized disease-management programs. A multidisciplinary approach to patient care is offered, in addition to diagnostic testing, extensive patient education, exercise programs, and nutritional counseling.

Digestive Diseases

Interest in specialized services for digestive diseases is a relatively new development for hospitals. It is estimated that 30 percent of visits to family practitioners are for digestive-related disorders.[15] Although this represents a unique market niche for ambulatory diversification, most hospitals have developed these units in order to prevent procedures from being initiated in freestanding facilities and physicians' offices. Some institutions have developed these services into organized programs simply because growth of procedures has far exceeded facility space. Generally, comprehensive digestive disease programs are multidisciplinary in nature. Services commonly offered include standard endoscopic procedures, such as colonoscopies and sigmoidoscopies, as well as such specific services as colorectal studies and treatment of incontinence disorders.

Pain Management

Similar to the specialized emphasis on disease disorders in ambulatory care settings, the concept of managing pain associated with these conditions is a new growth area for hospitals. Currently, chronic pain is estimated to exist in 40 million individuals; the cost of chronic pain is estimated to be $40 to $100 million annually.[16] Chronic intractable pain problems are generally defined as those that are unresponsive to traditional treatment. In one study, the average chronic pain patient had suffered for seven years, undergone three to five major operations, and spent $50,000 to $100,000 on medical bills.[17] Pain centers vary in their operation and approach to patient treatment. Generally, a multidisciplinary approach is utilized. The process involves comprehensive and exhaustive investigation into the many factors that may be responsible for the pain. Depending on the pain problems encountered, a number of therapeutic interventions can be used, including nerve blocks, transcutaneous nerve stimulation, biofeedback, acupuncture, hypnotherapy, psychotherapy, relaxation therapy, massage, and surgery. Despite criticisms of them, pain centers have been highly successful in treating patients; some programs indicate that 75 percent of patient treatments are successful. Payment for pain therapy in the outpatient setting is often identical to other traditional forms of outpatient reimbursement; however, some insurers do not reimburse for these services because of the lack of established standards. Some services, such as nerve blocks, rehabilitation, and psychological counseling, are inconsistently covered.

Sleep Disorders

It is estimated that approximately 30 percent of the population suffers from some form of sleep disorder, including sleep apnea (periods of breathlessness during the night in conjunction with loud snoring), insomnia (difficulty in falling asleep), and narcolepsy (uncontrollable sleepiness during the daytime).[18] Although sleep disorders can develop early in life, their incidence increases with age; many elderly persons suffer from sleep impairments. In general, formally organized sleep disorder programs perform diagnostic testing evaluations; patients then are referred to physician specialists for further treatment. For instance, sleep apnea patients can be referred to ear, nose, and throat or pulmonary specialists; insomnia patients can be referred to family practitioners and internists; and narcolepsy patients can be referred to neurologists.

The Future of Specialty Outpatient Care

Overall, developing specialized comprehensive outpatient programs, services, or "centers" for various disease disorders is a lengthy process. Continued technological change, provider acceptance, and recognition that highly specialized approaches to these disorders is effective will substantiate further ambulatory care growth. Decentralization of such programs will also allow for a more accurate definition of costs, thus allowing hospitals to offer services competitively.

Home Care

The implementation of the prospective payment system in 1983 and the continued advances in technology have created the impetus to deliver cost-effective care in the home environment. The prospective payment system has encouraged hospitals to discharge patients more quickly because it pays a flat rate for care based on a patient's diagnosis. By delivering care in the home setting, providers can reduce expenses by avoiding additional days of higher charges associated with inpatients.

Previously, home care was looked upon as an opportunity to not only reduce average length of stay, but also provide a new source of revenue through diversification. Although the former has been achieved, the latter is a subject of debate and widespread concern. Many hospitals have cited numerous problems in receiving reimbursement in a timely manner. Some claims are rejected without clear and concise reasons, and profit margins associated with the various home care segments have not lived up to expectations, particularly for Medicare beneficiaries.

Although many challenges exist, home care continues to experience moderate growth as an industry segment of a dynamic marketplace. It is projected that nearly $16 billion will be spent on home care by 1990.[19] Home care programs are a popular diversification strategy; over 40 percent are estimated to produce a positive bottom line, and 39 percent are at a break-even status.[20]

According to a survey conducted in 1986 by the Division of Ambulatory Care and Health Promotion of the American Hospital Association, 57 percent of hospitals provided home care services.[21] In addition, hospitals are rapidly diversifying into such areas as skilled care, home intravenous (IV) therapy, durable medical equipment, private pay services, and retail home care/pharmacy centers. This movement has occurred in spite of the previously mentioned challenges facing all providers. Today, a typical home care program provides approximately 8,000 Medicare visits, refers nearly 12 percent of total discharges to home care, is structured as a nonprofit operation, and has Medicare revenue as the largest source of all revenues.

It is interesting to note that Medicare-certified, hospital-based home care agencies represent the fastest-growing segment of the home care industry. Although the home care market is maturing, home care is no longer focusing on the elderly population alone. New areas of growth include psychiatric home care, early maternity care, well-born baby care, pediatric care, ambulatory surgery and emergency department follow-up, and care of occupational/industrial medicine patients.

In the future, hospitals will have to approach potential home care market segments with caution and with an understanding of the realistic financial expectations and the numerous barriers to entry. Increasingly, home care will become more heavily regulated with the advent of a prospective payment system, rigorous documentation requirements and utilization review by the federal government, and scrutiny of the quality of care operations and risk-management activities.

Occupational Health and Industrial Medicine

Of key diversification strategies in ambulatory care, occupational health/industrial medicine ranks second after women's health among all services that hospitals plan to offer in the future.[22] Until recently, these services traditionally have been provided through company-based employee health services or through employer contracts with freestanding clinics. Hospitals are now realizing that they are uniquely qualified to provide these services because they already have specialized medical resources and staff. These include the emergency department, laboratory, pharmacy, and resources for radiology, physical therapy, and inpatient care. When integrated with health education, substance abuse, and mental health facilities, the result can be a comprehensive service mix available from few other providers.

In essence, hospital-based occupational health programs provide several advantages to hospitals, including increased utilization of hospital services, increased referrals for hospital medical staff members, an enhanced opportunity to serve community health needs, and the fostering of a strong constituency among such influential groups as leaders from business and industry. In addition, approximately 3 to 4 admissions are generated per 100 occupational health visits, suggesting that a well-run occupational health program has the potential to increase a hospital's population base for admissions. Hospitals also find strong demand for their occupational health services by becoming health managers for businesses. By expanding their occupational health services to include claims processing, discharge planning, preadmission certification, and disability management, a comprehensive range of services can be provided for employers.

Of the 226 hospitals that provide occupational health services, the majority of programs are located in areas where the service population is between 100,000 and 2,500,000.[23] In contrast, only 18 percent of occupational/industrial medicine programs are offered in nonmetropolitan areas. In terms of location of service, 62 percent of hospitals operate services from one location; 16 percent are located in a freestanding building on a hospital campus; and 25 percent provide services in two locations.

Despite the relative newness of most occupational/industrial medicine programs, the services offered by most hospitals are extensive. As shown in table 2-2, the most frequently provided services are clinical, ancillary, industrial hygiene, consultative, educational, health promotion, and administrative. Although substantial growth is projected, occupational health/industrial medicine programs will face an increasing number of obstacles during their development. Resistance from medical staff members will continue to plague implementation; declining patient volume in physician offices will increase physicians' fear of additional competition in the marketplace. Besides physician resistance, problems will be encountered in developing, organizing, and promoting these programs. Unfortunately, the placement of these programs will differ by institution; the ideal organizational structure has yet to emerge.

Sports Medicine

Sports medicine programs are a new area of diversification for hospitals. The current preoccupation with physical fitness and endurance training has resulted in a marked increase in sports-related injuries and thus an opportunity to expand and increase market share of a new population segment.

Although the exact number of sports medicine programs provided by hospitals is unknown, a number of hospitals have indicated their intent to

Table 2-2. Occupational Health Services Most Frequently Provided by Hospitals, 1986

Service	Percentage
Clinical Services	
Periodic personal screening/evaluation for effects of workplace hazards	81.2
Preemployment physical examinations	76.8
Preplacement physical examinations	75.9
Diagnosis and treatment of work-related injuries and illnesses	75.0
Executive physical examinations	68.8
Ancillary Services	
Pulmonary function screening	80.4
Blood testing and laboratory services for toxicology	78.6
Audiometric testing to meet OSHA standards	76.8
Vision screening	76.8
Radiography	67.9
Immunizations	67.9
Screening for heavy metal exposure	62.5
Industrial Hygiene Services	
Environmental survey and inspection for worksite health hazards	58.0
Consultation on use of appropriate personal protective equipment	52.7
Toxic hazard information resources	47.3
Periodic personal or environmental toxic hazard monitoring	41.0
Consultative Services	
Consultation with management in development of policy/procedures	64.3
Evaluation of occupational health problems	64.3
Assistance in compliance with government health and safety regulations	58.9
Review of workers' compensation	52.7
Consultation on potential toxins in the workplace	45.5
Educational Services	
Back-injury risk reduction	83.0
CPR training	76.8
First-aid training	66.1
Information seminars for clients	60.7
Presentations by medical or administrative staff to outside medical and lay groups	57.1
Health Promotion Services	
Screening for specific disease risk	81.3
Screening for hypertension	78.6
Weight reduction	76.6
Stress management	74.1
Non–job-related health risk appraisal	72.3
Administrative Services	
Develop health care cost-containment strategies	36.6
Determine health-related cost of company	33.0
Design record-keeping systems	28.6
Provide physician representation during litigation	23.2
Evaluate benefit packages	17.0

Source: *Profile of Hospital Occupational Health Services.* Chicago: American Hospital Association, 1986.

develop this service. A 1986 survey conducted by the American Hospital Association's Division of Ambulatory Care and Health Promotion indicated that of 1,311 hospitals responding to the survey, approximately 80 percent said they were involved or getting involved in sports medicine. Some 24 percent indicated that they plan to offer a sports medicine program, and about one-third said they were considering the development of this program.

In addition, 25 percent already offered such programs. Only 20 percent said they had no interest in sports medicine. According to a separate survey, of those hospitals that offer sports medicine programs, nearly 43 percent are making money and 38 percent are breaking even on their operations.

Despite its popularity, sports medicine is still evolving and is often characterized as a rubric for programs with vast differences in personnel, organizational structure, and service offerings. Sports medicine programs range from small rooms with minimal exercise equipment to large, multidisciplinary programs comprised of numerous medical specialties and state-of-the-art fitness facilities. Hospitals contend that the programs generate inpatient admissions and are a good source of community public relations. Yet, as with other diversification programs, carefully defined goals and objectives must be developed in order to ensure a program's success. This is particularly important for hospitals considering sports medicine, for a number of industry critics contend that the market for these programs may have already plateaued.

Health Promotion

Health promotion is one area of the traditional domain of hospital service offerings that increasingly is being incorporated into the continuum of ambulatory care services. For many years, health promotion activities were considered to foster goodwill toward the hospital through community health education lectures, diagnostic screening, and information for hospital employees. Although many hospitals viewed these activities as necessary and appropriate, few could quantify savings through reduced health care utilization or achieve financial viability of the programs offered.

Today, however, health promotion is looked upon as a major component of the ambulatory process — to provide information, foster better understanding and compliance with treatment, teach new skills in self-management, encourage positive changes in life-style, and offer support and sometimes the setting in which those skills and new behaviors can be practiced. Health promotion will no doubt be a critical factor as hospitals increase cost-containment efforts, shifting more inpatients to the outpatient setting and decreasing costs for all outpatients when a prospective payment system is implemented in 1991.

The number of health promotion programs has remained constant from 1983 to 1987, and hospitals have shown a continued commitment to these programs. Integral to this process, patient education activities are receiving much attention. Patient education assists health promotion initiatives by shortening lengths of stay through early discharge planning to ambulatory care alternatives, by improving each patient's compliance with prescribed therapies, and by lessening the need for readmission and ambulatory care follow-up.

In the future, hospitals seeking a competitive edge in ambulatory care should incorporate health promotion and patient education activities to ensure a cost-effective delivery of patient care services. As more patients become knowledgeable about their illnesses and can participate in these decisions, movement to ambulatory care programs can be enhanced. And, if ambulatory care is to be successful, these initiatives will have to become an important part of the patient care process.

Behavioral Medicine

Behavioral medicine, which consists of psychiatric and chemical dependency services, represents yet another area of hospital diversification in ambulatory care. This trend is significant; the annual cost of behavioral health services exceeds $100 billion annually, and alcohol and drug abuse add $27 billion to the cost of health insurance.[24]

Despite employee cost sharing, hospital preauthorization, and the prospective payment system, major payers are witnessing double-digit increases in their behavioral health costs. In the early 1980s, many businesses liberalized health benefits for behavioral problems; now they face increases of over 20 percent in their health plan costs for these services. Because major employers and other providers opt for this care, reimbursement increasingly is being scrutinized by them. This will create tremendous opportunities for ambulatory care providers as they seek to cut inpatient stays, shift to more appropriate settings, and develop risk-sharing contracting arrangements.

In 1987, 1,416 hospitals (22.5 percent) indicated that they provide alcoholism/chemical dependency outpatient services.[25] This represents an increase of 107 percent over the 684 programs in 1983. Almost the same percentages were reported for psychiatric outpatient services during this period. These data reveal an area of opportunity for hospitals. One estimate indicates that profit margins associated with these programs can range as high as 30 percent. Because some programs have shown that up to 65 percent of behavioral patients can be managed entirely within the ambulatory care environment, diversification in this arena must be carefully evaluated and implemented by hospitals.[26]

Observation Units

Although many ambulatory care approaches have emphasized freestanding programs, attention is now being directed at various hospital alternatives, especially observation units, which are viewed as an option to reduce routine hospital admissions or to prevent premature emergency department discharges.

Generally, there are three types of observation units: a designated area within the hospital emergency department, a designated area or "holding unit" in another hospital outpatient setting, and a specially designated inpatient area. Historically, emergency departments have been the domain of observation units; the other types of observation units have appeared only recently. Patients who are candidates for these units often are those needing observation subsequent to diagnostic testing, treatments, or surgery, or those awaiting admission, discharge, or transfer to another facility.

Observation units allow hospitals to reduce inappropriate admissions, enhance patient disposition and transfer, and provide continuous patient care at a low cost. Because patient charges are reimbursed as outpatient visits rather than inpatient admissions, the savings can be dramatic.

Observation Units in Emergency Departments

In the emergency department, a properly operated observation unit can enhance the medical care delivered, because additional time is given to patients who require more extensive observation following treatment. According to the American College of Emergency Physicians (ACEP) in Dallas, patients admitted to observation units should fall into one of two categories: (1) patients who are not expected to be hospitalized and who have a reasonable probability of discharge within a given time period; and (2) patients who require a prolonged period of observation or testing before a decision to admit or discharge is made. Patients with specific medical conditions who may be candidates for prolonged observation include those with asthma, allergic reactions, minor concussions, certain drug overdoses, mild alcohol intoxication, and specific toxic inhalations.

To ensure the successful operation of an observation/holding unit, well-documented policies and procedures are necessary. For instance, most emergency department units have a time limit of 12 hours for observing a patient before the patient's disposition is finalized. Often, however, this time period can reach almost 24 hours.

Thus, it is imperative that the responsibility of the observation unit be clearly defined. Generally, in the emergency department setting, the emergency department physician should assume care of the patient until the patient is admitted or the patient's private physician assumes management of the patient. In addition, the unit should be staffed by at least one nurse who is permanently assigned to the area, in order to ensure that staff members are familiar with the unit's philosophy, goals, policies, and procedures.

Holding Units

Holding units differ from observation units in that patients are treated in a separate outpatient area and fall into one of two categories: (1) those patients requiring specialized outpatient therapy, such as intravenous antibiotic therapy, chemotherapy, and the like; and (2) those awaiting either transfer from the hospital to another facility or an inpatient bed.

Holding units are particularly useful because patients who formerly required hospitalization can now receive diagnostic/therapeutic regimens on an outpatient basis, thus eliminating higher charges and improving patient satisfaction. More important, holding units maximize the ability of staff members outside the holding unit to assist other emergency department patients.

Guidelines for a holding unit are similar to those for an emergency department observation unit, with properly defined admission criteria, policies and procedures, staffing, equipment, and quality assistance review. Because of the varied nature of the outpatients who may utilize the holding unit, it is particularly important that policies and staffing be appropriate for unique patient needs, such as reactions to infrequently used treatments, allergic reactions, the differing treatment protocols of various physicians, and so forth. In addition, this area may be involved in the transfer or acceptance of patients to or from other facilities, as outlined in the 1986 COBRA guidelines. Adequate documentation and knowledge of transfer policies are particularly important as they relate to these guidelines.

Extended Observation Beds

Since the passage of the prospective payment system, an extension of the 12-hour observation unit has been created. Commonly referred to as 23-hour observation beds, these extended observation beds allow Medicare patients to be admitted for up to but not exceeding 24 hours. Because hospitals are not reimbursed for Medicare admissions that are determined to be unnecessary, the observation unit clearly meets an important need. These beds provide an area to care for patients who do not meet criteria for hospitalization, but do have conditions that require an extended period of observation. In addition, the beds can be used for other purposes, such as for outpatient surgical patients who may require additional observation prior to discharge.

Women's Health Care

Organized, comprehensive programs aimed at women have received much attention from hospitals in the past few years. In 1986, women's health care services were ranked as the top diversification strategy in a survey conducted by the American Hospital Association's Division of Ambulatory Care and Health Promotion. In 1987, 752 hospitals, or 12.5 percent of 6,281 U.S. hospitals, indicated that they operated some form of women's health programs. In a survey of women's programs in operation in 1987, nearly 50 percent were making money, and nearly 30 percent were operating at a break-even status.

Several factors support the interest in and growth of these centers: women make 80 percent of health care decisions for their families; women are the largest utilizers of preventive services and health promotion programs; and women use far more health services than men do each year. Initial women's health programs focused on obstetrical and gynecological services. They have since evolved to include a multidisciplinary array of service offerings. Today, typical programs offer medical services ranging from well visits to treatment of major illnesses, psychotherapy, nutritional counseling, mammography screening, support groups, and a number of educational programs related to women's health issues. Some programs have incorporated fitness evaluations, genetic counseling, weight-loss and smoking-cessation programs, and self-referral programs.

The success enjoyed by some programs is the result of careful market research of women's specific health care needs. Generally, women prefer to have a wide array of services available to them, such as one-stop shopping, in convenient and comfortable settings. The strong consumer orientation of most women's health programs appears to be the motivating factor for their acceptance by women. Their acceptance also attests to the impact that a strong consumer orientation can have on other ambulatory care programs and services.

Challenges Created by Ambulatory Care Growth

The previous discussions of the magnitude of ambulatory care growth and the resulting revenues from the multitude of services offered portray a scenario of success for many hospitals and providers. Yet, accompanying this growth are many diverse and complex challenges that must be confronted by hospitals. These include coping with the impending reform of Medicare Part B reimbursement, adjusting to cost-containment initiatives by other third parties, conducting productivity assessment and enhancement, ensuring quality of care validation, responding to an increasingly changing patient mix, and developing and managing information capabilities to care for ambulatory patients.

Medicare Outpatient Reimbursement

Among the health care services covered by Medicare, reimbursement for hospital outpatient services has shown the largest rate of growth. With the advent of the prospective payment system, hospital outpatient expenditures have increased phenomenally. In 1987, Medicare charges for hospital outpatient services amounted to $9.6 billion—an increase of 256 percent over $2.7 billion in 1983.[27] Similarly, the average outpatient reimbursement per enrollee has grown from $92 in 1983 to $136 in 1985—an increase of almost 50 percent.

The prospective payment system has created incentives for hospitals to hold down costs because they earn a profit when their costs fall below the prospective payment and absorb a loss when their costs exceed the payment threshold. As a result, providers have been shortening lengths of stay, reducing ancillary services, and fostering outpatient alternatives for care. According to an interim report on the impact of prospective payment on hospitals, preliminary findings indicate reasons why ambulatory care is one of the fastest-growing segments of the health care industry: (1) there are direct financial incentives for hospitals to shift care to ambulatory settings when it is clinically appropriate and cost-efficient; (2) surgical and diagnostic innovations have enabled hospitals to perform more procedures on an ambulatory basis; (3) utilization review policies have influenced the Medicare patient mix in hospitals, because preadmission review now encourages treatment in the most appropriate and cost-effective setting; and (4) the addition of ambulatory surgical benefits and the repeal of the deductible for home health services have encouraged greater outpatient use.

As discussed earlier, HCFA has long recognized the need to create further incentives for efficiency and productivity. It appears that the early 1990s will be the beginning of payment reform for all ambulatory care services. A number of payment initiatives have been studied, but a specific patient classification has yet to be endorsed or demonstrated in a full-scale system implementation.

Industry Cost-Containment Initiatives

In 1987, spending for the nation's health care services reached $500 billion. As a percentage of the gross national product (GNP), expenditures reached 11.1 percent in 1987, up from 10.7 percent in 1986 and almost double the percentage in 1965. By the year 2000, HCFA predicts that health spending will represent 15 percent of the GNP.[28] There are numerous reasons for the explosive growth in health care costs, and attention is now being focused on every effort to contain these expenditures.

Currently, two-thirds of health care provided in the United States is funded by employers via insurance benefits to employees.[29] In order to stem the increases in costs, many employers are offering their employees incentives to use services other than inpatient services, or in some cases are demanding that outpatient alternatives be used exclusively. Because as a group employers represent one of the major buyers of health care services, their influence in determining what services will be utilized is significant. They are becoming more sophisticated in purchasing and evaluating health care services.

Although companies provide coverage for outpatient alternatives, the majority of companies continue to reimburse employees for these services at the same rate as inpatient care. This trend alone is mainly responsible for the claim that outpatient care, although appropriate, is not a less costly alternative to inpatient services. Companies are, however, attempting to ensure that expenditures are warranted. Over 90 percent of companies now require mandatory second opinions for surgical care or offer financial incentives to employees who obtain second opinions on their own behalf.[30]

In addition to certain changes in health benefit design plans, a number of companies now require mandatory cost sharing from employees who utilize certain health care services. Most companies require employees to pay 20 percent of charges for most services subject to a copayment.[31] Copayments, premiums, and deductibles are other forms of employee cost sharing that are increasingly being utilized by employers.

In recent years, industry has embraced the concept that in order to reduce health care expenditures, utilization of services must be controlled. Thus the concept of "managed care" has evolved, and many companies, insurers, and payers have implemented various managed care protocols. In terms of providing ambulatory care services, preservice certification requirements will allow early payer intervention in elective ambulatory services, identifying those patients whose condition could be unusually expensive or more expensive than anticipated or require a greater intensity of follow-up care.

Productivity Assessment

The assessment and management of productivity in the ambulatory care setting will be difficult for hospitals in the 1990s. Because ambulatory care is provided to numerous patients and often involves multiple procedures performed in various departments or settings, it is highly labor-intensive. And, because ambulatory care services have low profit margins per unit of service, it is difficult to maintain overall program viability because the level of services performed often exceeds the level of available resources.

To achieve the critical balance between improved productivity and high-quality patient care in the ambulatory setting, hospitals will have to adopt a number of innovative strategies. First, hospital management will have to embrace a broad set of goals and policies for ambulatory care delivery. These measures will determine to a great extent the efficiency and effectiveness with which each institution can organize resources to deliver and manage ambulatory care patients. Second, productivity management programs will need to be implemented to ensure that various services are delivered to ambulatory patients on a clinically justified basis, as well as in the most appropriate and cost-effective manner. Finally, operational efficiency must be achieved through high-level managerial development. To achieve such operational productivity, the development of support systems that allow employees to attain their full working potential must be initiated.

Because productivity standards are now viewed as crucial variables in the delivery of ambulatory care, adherence to these measures will determine the ultimate success of each ambulatory program or service. Once ambulatory growth stabilizes and revenue maximization is achieved, the only viable option to improve operational effectiveness will be cost reduction through productivity improvement.

Defining Quality of Service

Despite the constant debate as to what variables constitute an accurate definition of high quality in delivery of health care services, greater attention to quality issues in the ambulatory setting will be exercised by various providers. This is a formidable task because systematic review of outpatients is difficult to achieve. For instance, the large volume of patients treated in ambulatory settings does not lend itself to total review of all patients; treatment outcomes may be difficult to ascertain; medical record charting is often incomplete and noncomputerized; and the review process is often very subjective in terms of factors contributing to a patient's outcome.

Because determining the quality of patient care is both subjective and objective in nature, a definition of high quality in ambulatory care delivery will no doubt include all of these parameters. The Quality Assurance Committee of the Society for Ambulatory Care Professionals, a personal membership organization of the American Hospital Association, contends that levels of quality in the ambulatory care setting equal the attributes associated with that care. Thus, attributes of high-quality health care can be measured in such a way as to demonstrate the positive level of quality. Each attribute of high-quality care is one that a reasonable purchaser of health care associates with good quality and expects to have provided. To this end, attributes include the effectiveness of care delivered or technical competency; the acceptability of services; access to or the availability of services; consideration of the value-added concept; and continuity of care.

The movement toward defining and measuring quality will also create challenges for hospitals in terms of how level of quality relates to profits. Increasingly, payers are adopting the philosophy that high-quality care costs much less in the long term than lower-quality care. High-quality care reduces the costs incurred by low-quality care. For example, when the quality of care is high, less is spent on inspection, maintenance, and replacement of technology; and a higher-quality product or service may increase the possibility of charging a higher price for a valued service. Thus, high quality of services can actually cost less and generate higher profits. Particularly in the ambulatory care arena, where services are more price-sensitive than in the inpatient setting, hospitals must continually enhance their quality of care assessments if they wish to remain strong competitors in the health care marketplace.

Changing Patient Mix

A number of forces are currently changing the patient mix, challenging the health care industry's ability to meet the demands of specific population segments. The tremendous increase in the number of AIDS patients and the increased prevalence of disease among the aged, the homeless, and the uninsured and underinsured pose serious problems for providers. Ambulatory care settings will be most affected, because the initial and sometimes only points of entry into the health care system for these patients are emergency departments and community health centers. Home care programs, for instance, are the treatment location of choice for patients with AIDS or chronic illnesses. As these patients multiply in number and the population ages, the service capacity necessary to care for all patients will be strained and the profitability of overall operations will be questionable for some institutions.

The fundamental shift from inpatient to outpatient is also creating a new category of ambulatory patients that was not seen five years ago. Generally, these patients have very complex medical problems, and they may be dependent on sophisticated technological equipment on a daily basis. While undergoing ambulatory procedures or testing, they require more preparation time, more transportation time, and more supervision by nursing and technical personnel. Thus, the mix of these patients in ambulatory settings will create challenges to achieving productivity standards and operational efficiency targets.

Management Information Needs

Meeting management information needs will provide a challenge to hospitals in the 1990s and beyond. Increasing pressures are being placed on hospitals and other providers to develop comprehensive, integrated outpatient data bases for all ambulatory care programs. The federal government's intent to create a fully prospective payment system for all outpatients by 1991 is a major force behind this movement; however, it also is being fueled by the growth of alternative delivery systems, competitors, and other structural changes in the health care system.

Currently, it is acknowledged that tremendous amounts of data exist for ambulatory care services; however, their usefulness is limited because of a lack of standard definitions, a lack of clinical/financial integration, and a lack of systems available from information system vendors. Interest in the demand for ambulatory care data has existed for some time, and the lack of such information is attributed largely to the lack of a uniform data set for units of service that are provided in ambulatory settings.

In addition, ambulatory care providers use a wide variety of coding conventions and coding languages. Although the Current Procedural Terminology (CPT-4) coding system is becoming more prevalent as a result of recent federal legislative initiatives, many institutions have found using it to be a cumbersome and painful exercise. Previously, almost all ambulatory care data had been compiled manually and then was stored for a specific data reporting purpose; it was therefore often unusable for new and different data tasks.

As hospitals begin to evaluate operational changes to accommodate the medical records, billing, information systems, and other requirements in this new health care environment, they must capture the requisite clinical and financial data and provide a means to measure productivity and ensure efficiency in managing patient care. Unless this is done, some providers will find themselves at a great disadvantage in trying to achieve a competitive edge in ambulatory care service delivery.

Issues Specific to Various Hospitals

Although ambulatory care development and expansion will be challenged by many environmental forces, as was detailed in the previous discussion, a number of hospitals will face unique issues because of their specific role and orientation. They include, but are not limited to, teaching hospitals and tertiary care facilities, community hospitals, and small or rural facilities. Because they differ in many respects, such as demographics of patients served, services offered, and mix of medical staff members, their responses to the new health care environment will not be uniform.

Teaching and Tertiary Care Hospitals

Historically, teaching and tertiary care hospitals have not considered ambulatory care services a priority. Still, many have been involved extensively in ambulatory care via numerous primary care clinics and faculty practice plans. Because the shift to ambulatory care has caused a dramatic decrease in the number of patients admitted to these institutions, outpatient care is now a survival strategy for them.

A number of issues affect the role and mission of teaching institutions in the delivery of ambulatory care services. Their traditional emphasis on education and research, for instance, is difficult to maintain in the new era of ambulatory care delivery, because additional costs must be incurred along with funding for inpatient-related activities. In addition, to remain competitive with other providers, these institutions will have to reorganize their current structures to attain a more appropriate balance of primary care physicians, and specialists and delivery sites. Perhaps most important, teaching hospitals that wish to attract ambulatory care patients will have to be competitive in terms of price, quality, and service. Recent examples of these efforts are those institutions that have abolished clinic operations in favor of privatized medical group practice arrangements.

Community Hospitals

Short-term community hospitals have long been considered the prime developers of ambulatory care services. In communities with two or more institutions, competition has been strong to continually add new technology, programs, and services. Often, however, these services have caused unnecessary duplication between hospitals, causing severe underutilization of programs and financial losses. In addition, other expansion in communities by entrepreneurs and for-profit entities has further eroded each hospital's ability to maintain and increase market share.

Unfortunately, many short-term community hospitals that have the ability to expand ambulatory care services have been hindered by the concerns of their medical staff. Because physicians have delivered the majority of ambulatory-related services in communities, they have been skeptical of hospital ambulatory care development. Physicians have feared that these new endeavors will encroach on their practices and their income. Without the commitment of medical staff members, hospitals cannot be successful in the long-term provision of ambulatory care services. To minimize this conflict, physicians increasingly must be made integral members in all stages of ambulatory care development.

Small or Rural Hospitals

Of the 5,611 community hospitals in 1987, 2,599, or nearly 50 percent, were small or rural institutions. Despite their size or geographic location, small or rural hospitals have been responsible for a large portion of the total ambulatory care growth increases in the past few years. This is largely because these facilities have only recently begun to develop ambulatory care expansion efforts. For instance, in 1983 only 737 small or rural hospitals had organized outpatient departments, versus 1,397 in 1987 — an increase of 90 percent.[32] In addition, in 1983 only 24 percent of total surgeries were performed on an outpatient basis in these facilities, versus 42 percent in 1987 — an increase of 75 percent.

The push to outpatient care in small or rural hospitals comes at a time when the financial viability of many facilities is of great concern. During 1986 and 1987 alone, 160 small or rural facilities closed in the United States. In the future, additional closings of small or rural facilities will require innovative solutions to ensure access to health care both for inpatients and outpatients. If a hospital must close, one strategy may be to develop a freestanding ambulatory care facility that offers 24-hour emergency care, observation beds for extended patient care (up to 72 hours), subsequent discharge or transfer to another institution, and onsite physician offices for the delivery of primary medical care. For those facilities that remain operational, future ambulatory care expansion increasingly will be conducted both with existing medical staff members and via joint venture arrangements with neighboring institutions and regional referral centers. Because access to capital and state-of-the-art technology will be difficult, ambulatory care developments may arise only through carefully planned and directed efforts with parties that share similar interests.

Moving toward Integration

The changing delivery structure of the health care system will test each health care facility's ability to compete effectively with multiple providers in matured markets. As ambulatory care is accepted as a significant force in the patient care process, hospitals will make large commitments to integrate ambulatory care services and to become formidable players in ambulatory care delivery. Because current patient flow problems will continue to exacerbate due to inadequate space capacity to treat all patients, greater demand for diagnostic testing and services, and increased acuity of patients, total reorganization of ambulatory care services and programs will be necessary.

To this end, current ambulatory care programs and services will be enhanced or deleted; new programs will evolve based upon institutional commitment and marketplace needs; and services that were once predominantly inpatient will be performed only in outpatient settings. Ambulatory care services will occur in a multitude of facility settings. Various ambulatory care services will be provided in hospital-based settings; some will be done in freestanding and mobile units; and some will be provided exclusively in each of these settings. The integration of all ambulatory care programs and services will be a goal for many institutions; the achievement of that goal will be a factor that will ultimately determine an institution's long-term survival.

References

1. Matson, T. A. The explosive growth of ambulatory care: challenges and opportunities for hospitals. Presentation, Evangelical Health Systems, Good Shepherd Hospital, Barrington, IL, Nov. 20, 1986.

2. Matson, T. A. Rethinking the delivery of ambulatory care: hospital-based versus freestanding alternatives. Presentation, "Penetrating the Alternative Site Market-

place Conference," Biomedical Business International, San Francisco, Sept. 15, 1987.

3. Matson, T. A. The hospital emergency department in transition. Presentation, "The Hospital Emergency Department: Returning to Financial Viability Conference," American Hospital Association, Chicago, July 16, 1986.

4. Matson, Rethinking the delivery of ambulatory care.

5. Ambulatory care growth continues. *Outreach* 10(1):2, Jan.–Feb. 1989.

6. Ambulatory care growth continues, p. 2.

7. Biomedical Business International. *Clinical Laboratory Services Industry.* BBI report no. 7076. Tustin, CA: BBI, 1987.

8. Biomedical Business International.

9. Biomedical Business International.

10. Nathanson, S. N., and Lerman, D. *Outpatient Cancer Centers: Implementation and Management.* Chicago: American Hospital Publishing, 1988.

11. Personal communication. National Head Injury Foundation. Framingham, MA, Mar. 1989.

12. Souhrada, L. Hospitals consider allergy and asthma programs. *Hospitals* 62(16):84, Aug. 20, 1988.

13. Personal communication. Arthritis Foundation. Atlanta, Mar. 1989.

14. Personal communication. American Diabetes Association. Alexandria, VA, Apr. 1989.

15. Division of Health Care Statistics. *The National Ambulatory Medical Care Survey.* Washington, DC: National Center for Health Statistics, 1979.

16. East Central Michigan Health Systems Agency. *A Report on the Task Force on Pain Centers.* Saginaw, MI: ECMHSA, 1978.

17. East Central Michigan Health Systems Agency.

18. Wingate, N. Sleep centers both consumer and physician driven. *Hospital Product Line Report* 2(7):9, Jan. 1988. Washington, DC: St. Anthony Hospital Publications.

19. Frost and Sullivan. *Home Healthcare Products and Services: Markets in the U.S.* New York City: Frost and Sullivan, 1983.

20. Sabatino, F. G. The diversification success story continues: survey. *Hospitals* 63(1):26, Jan. 5, 1989.

21. American Hospital Association, Division of Ambulatory Care and Health Promotion. *Home Care Survey.* Chicago: AHA, 1986.

22. American Hospital Association, *Home Care Survey.*

23. Hospitals enter occupational health arena. *Outreach* 8(2):1, Mar.–Apr. 1987.

24. National Institute on Alcohol Abuse and Alcoholism. *Characteristics of Alcoholism Services in the United States, 1984.* Washington, DC: NIAAA, 1986.

25. American Hospital Association. Table 12A. *Hospital Statistics, 1988 ed.* Chicago: AHA, 1988.

26. U.S. Department of Health and Human Services, National Institute of Mental Health. *Specialty Mental Health Organizations, United States 1983 to 1984.* Washington, DC: USDHHS, 1986.

27. Personal communication. U.S. Department of Health and Human Services, Health Care Financing Administration, Office of Research and Communications. Washington, DC, Jan. 1989.

28. National health expenditures, 1987. *Health Care Financing Review,* Winter 1988, p. 128.

29. *The Business Roundtable Health, Welfare, and Retirement Income Task Force Report: Corporate Health-Care-Cost Management and Private Sector Initiatives.* Indianapolis: The Business Roundtable, 1987.

30. The Business Roundtable Health, Welfare, and Retirement Income Task Force Report.

31. The Business Roundtable Health, Welfare, and Retirement Income Task Force Report.

32. American Hospital Association, Table 12A, *Hospital Statistics, 1988.*

Chapter 3

Legal Aspects of Reorganizing Ambulatory Care Capacity

Douglas M. Mancino

As discussed elsewhere in this book, hospitals are utilizing several different approaches to reorganizing their ambulatory care services. One approach is to consolidate and "repackage" existing programs and services into new product lines that have a clearer identity and are more marketable. Another approach is to establish new ambulatory care programs to meet particular demands or to take advantage of market opportunities. From a legal standpoint, however, a hospital typically may take one of three approaches. First, the hospital may reorganize existing ambulatory care programs or establish new ones within the legal entity that owns and operates the hospital itself. Second, the hospital may establish a new entity to take over existing ambulatory care programs or to establish new programs or departments. Third, the hospital may choose to involve physicians or other health care professionals on some form of risk-sharing basis in delivering ambulatory care programs and services. In this last case, the approach typically selected will be some form of a joint venture.

Regardless of which of the three approaches is selected, the hospital choosing to reorganize existing programs or establish new ambulatory care programs should address the legal considerations from strategic as well as from transactional perspectives. Obviously, the legal structure must fit the particular framework, whether it is a joint venture or a reorganization of existing programs, but it must also fit the strategy for that service.

In this chapter, we will explore some of the basic legal issues that will arise in connection with all three approaches.

Reorganizing Services within the Existing Corporate Structure

When a hospital wishes to reorganize existing ambulatory care programs or establish new capacity within its existing corporate structure, it will generally have to address many of the same legal issues that arise when restructuring or adding any other type of hospital service. However, the legal issues often will become more complicated than was originally expected because of some practical realities of ambulatory care program development. Some of these are basic and some are more esoteric. The key issues are discussed in this section.

Certificate of Need

Legislation in many states requires a certificate of need (CON) permit to establish or substantially expand certain types of health care facilities or services. Typically, the required approval granted by the health planning agency in response to the provider's application will be based on various criteria, such as need, financial feasibility, impact on other health care providers, and access by indigents to the proposed services. Even though health planning and capital expenditure regulation have been undergoing dramatic changes throughout the United States during the past five years, and many states have repealed, allowed to expire, or reduced the scope of their CON laws, the CON laws still remain an important hurdle to be overcome in many states, particularly in the Northeast, Midwest, and Southeast.

In most states with CON laws, for example, a CON will be required if a hospital wishes to establish and operate a freestanding ambulatory surgery center. This type of project typically will be regarded as involving an expansion of outpatient surgical capacity, thereby requiring a CON. Similarly, the establishment of other types of ambulatory care programs, such as home health agencies and urgent care centers, may require a CON under the laws of the particular jurisdiction.

When a hospital wishes to establish an ambulatory care program that might require a CON, it should nevertheless explore whether other alternatives for avoidance of the CON requirements are available if it wishes to reduce the time or cost of establishing the program. For example, a number of states exempt from CON requirements activities that are conducted as part of a doctor's office. Thus, in the case of a freestanding ambulatory surgery center, it may be possible to structure a legal and operational relationship with a physician or group of physicians that will enable the ambulatory surgery center to be treated as part of a doctor's office for CON purposes, rather than as a hospital program. Similarly, diagnostic imaging centers, urgent care centers, and other ambulatory services that require significant physician involvement and participation may be capable of being structured under the doctor's office exemption.

Obviously, an examination of the laws of the particular state will be necessary to determine what types of ambulatory care services require a CON, whether a freestanding ambulatory surgery center must be licensed and must obtain a CON before receiving a license, whether the repositioning of existing ambulatory care services might trigger a CON requirement (perhaps, for example, because additional capital expenditures may be required), and what exemptions from CON requirements may be available.

Licensing Considerations

State licensing statutes generally regulate the character and competence of the health provider and its staff, its financial resources, the fitness and adequacy of the facility, its medical or technical personnel, and its procedures. State licensing laws must always be examined to determine whether licensure may be required, may be obtained even if not required, or may be totally unavailable for the particular program or service.

If a license is required by state law, obtaining a separate license or adding the service to the hospital's existing license may be necessary in order to receive payment under certain types of payment and reimbursement programs. Nevertheless, there may be some unique consequences of licensure that will have to be taken into account in determining whether licensure is available and, even if it is, whether it should be pursued.

One important licensing-related issue is the potential applicability of hospital building and life safety codes to an activity that is included as an outpatient department of the hospital. In some states, classification of an ambulatory care program as an outpatient department of the hospital will entail significantly greater building costs to comply with the building, safety, and other requirements generally applicable to hospitals. If this is the case, then the ambulatory care program may be placed at a competitive disadvantage by the increased costs of compliance. On the other hand, other states, such as California, have amended licensing and building standards to "level the playing field" for ambulatory care services conducted by hospitals by mandating that building, life safety, and other requirements for such ambulatory services be no greater than those applicable to freestanding facilities that perform similar services. If such relief is not available, the hospital should consider whether it is possible to structure the activity to avoid hospital licensing requirements without adversely affecting its reimbursement or other operational objectives.

Another consideration affected by licensure may be the geographic location of the outpatient department. Some states may condition licensure as an outpatient department of the hospital upon the location of the ambulatory care program within the hospital premises or on the hospital campus. By contrast, other states, such as California, permit the licensure of off-campus remote hospital outpatient departments, provided that the hospital exercises sufficient control over them.

Tax Considerations

If the sponsor of the ambulatory care program is a not-for-profit, tax-exempt hospital, it will need to evaluate the program in light of the income tax exemption requirements applicable to tax-exempt hospitals. In general, any program conducted by a hospital will be regarded as a separate trade or business for federal income tax purposes. As a consequence, some ambulatory care programs may be free from taxation, whereas others may be taxable.

For example, if a hospital establishes a freestanding ambulatory surgery center, the revenues derived from the operation of that center should be free from business income tax. The reason for this tax-free treatment is that the operation of an ambulatory surgery center generally promotes the health of the community in a charitable sense, as long as its access is limited to a small segment of the community. Thus, it may be enough for the ambulatory surgery center to become a Medicare-certified provider (assuming it is not operated as a hospital-based surgery center) in order to obtain tax-free status for its revenues. Similar treatment should be available for a home health agency that operates as a Medicare provider.

On the other hand, sales and leases of durable medical equipment may constitute taxable activities, especially if they are not carried on primarily for the convenience of the hospital's inpatients or outpatients. For example, the establishment of a durable medical equipment supply business by an otherwise tax-exempt hospital may be a taxable activity.

Other Practical Legal Considerations

As hospitals develop and expand ambulatory care capacity, they also must anticipate and address a variety of practical legal considerations. For example, prior to embarking on any expanded or new ambulatory care program, the hospital should undertake a review of its contracts with its hospital-based physicians to check for potential conflict of interest. For example, hospital-based physician contracts in certain departments, such as radiology, pathology, and emergency, often contain exclusivity requirements and non-competition covenants. The exclusivity requirements may require the hospital to employ the physician group under contract for its ambulatory care activity, even if the hospital wishes to establish an ambulatory care program in a location away from the main hospital campus that does not directly compete with the hospital's program. In addition, hospital-based physician contracts typically contain provisions dealing with the pricing of the professional components of the ambulatory care service. Again, these clauses may reduce the hospital's ability to meet competition if the pricing policies in the ambulatory care setting must be tied to the pricing policies in the inpatient setting.

Another legal consideration involves the various accreditation requirements applicable to the ambulatory care activities. A decision needs to be made as to whether the hospital desires the hospital-based ambulatory care program to be treated for accreditation purposes as a hospital-based or a freestanding program. This decision may affect the accreditation standards applicable to the activity.

The hospital must also address the credentialing, quality assurance, and risk management aspects of the ambulatory care activity. These issues, unfortunately, are not well developed in the statutory or case law. Nevertheless, such issues as confidentiality of medical staff disciplinary proceedings are of great significance and can be affected by the way in which the ambulatory care program is structured.

Operating Ambulatory Care Programs through Separate Corporations

There may be several reasons why ambulatory care programs should be conducted by separate corporations. For example, operating the ambulatory care program through a separate corporation may facilitate avoidance of CON requirements otherwise applicable to the hospital or may facilitate treatment of the ambulatory care program as a freestanding program for reimbursement or accreditation purposes. In addition, operation of an ambulatory care program through a separate entity may reduce liability risks for malpractice and other types of catastrophic financial exposure. Finally, there may be management, financial, or other legal reasons that warrant the operation of the ambulatory care program through one or more separate corporations.

Designing the Right Corporate Structure

There is no "right" corporate structure that will be applicable to every situation. A hospital should not establish a new corporation or reorganize an existing corporation as an end in and of itself. Rather, the form through which the ambulatory care program is conducted should be suited to the particular needs of that program.

Figure 3-1 is a depiction of the typical parent–subsidiary corporate structure for new health care systems. Under this structure, the parent corporation (whether investor-owned or not-for-profit) is responsible for strategic direction, allocation of financial resources, and management of the individual subsidiaries. The subsidiaries are, themselves, responsible for day-to-day operations of their respective businesses. The hierarchical structure helps ensure that ultimate control is retained by the parent corporation through its ability to select or remove the directors or key management of the subsidiaries and through its ability to control allocation of financial and other resources.

Taxation of a New Corporation

For not-for-profit hospitals and health care systems, taxation is a key issue that needs to be addressed whenever a new corporation is formed: will tax-exempt status be available for the subsidiary? Some activities, such as

Figure 3-1. New Health Care System Structure

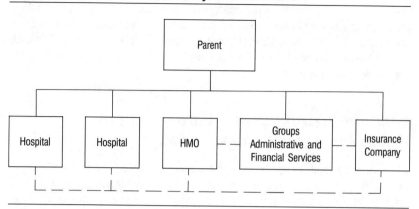

Source: McDermott, Will and Emery, Los Angeles, California, 1987.

ambulatory surgery centers and home health agencies, should readily qualify for tax-exempt status as separate entities as long as they are structured and operated to ensure that their facilities or services are reasonably accessible to the communities they are structured to serve. On the other hand, certain types of activities, such as diagnostic centers, high-risk obesity clinics, and primary care centers, may be structured in such a way as to closely resemble physicians' offices. In effect, then, to the extent that the ambulatory care activity is conducted by a separate corporation in a manner that looks more like a physician's office than it does a hospital-type service, the availability of tax-exempt status may be diminished.

Certificate of Need Requirements

Even if the ambulatory care program is conducted by a separate corporation, an examination of applicable CON requirements must be undertaken. For example, activities carried on by a hospital through a separate entity may nevertheless be regarded as being carried on "by or on behalf of" the hospital and thus may subject the separate entity to CON requirements. Conversely, when a hospital appears exempt from CON requirements, such as when it establishes an ambulatory surgery center with no expansion of surgical capacity, the ambulatory surgery center may not be applicable for a separate entity. Thus, these sorts of issues need to be addressed when one begins to consider whether to conduct the activities through a separate corporation.

Practical Licensing Problems

As indicated previously, licensure may be important to a particular program if reimbursement for the facility component of services is predicated on the availability of licensure. Thus, the issue of whether an activity must or should be separately incorporated can only be addressed correctly if the operational and financial ramifications of the separate corporation are considered. For example, if a hospital desires to operate a comprehensive cancer center, it may structure the center to function as an outpatient department of the hospital or as a physician's office. However, it is likely that no separate licensure may be available or required for such a comprehensive outpatient cancer center if it is owned and operated by a separate corporation.

Joint Ventures

During the past five years, the number of joint ventures used to develop and operate ambulatory care facilities and services has grown dramatically. The proliferation of ambulatory care joint ventures has had many causes. Perhaps most obvious are the new technological developments and financial incentives that have shifted the emphasis from inpatient care to outpatient care. Another cause is the growing numbers of physician–entrepreneurs who are seeking new sources of revenue at a time when the availability of new technologies, such as magnetic resonance imaging (MRI), has been improved and the need to supplement practice revenue has increased.

Another reason for the growth of joint ventures has been the role played by proprietary and investor-owned companies that specialize in the development and operation of ambulatory care facilities and services. These companies have galvanized hospital and physician support and provided financing for the development of ambulatory care facilities, such as freestanding surgery centers and diagnostic centers. The entry into the marketplace and the growth in numbers of these types of companies have helped accelerate the growth and demand for joint ventures in unexpected ways.

As the number of joint ventures has grown, so has the wealth of literature available to hospitals, physicians, and others seeking to establish one or more joint ventures.[1] This section will explore many of the issues and questions that typically must be addressed when developing a strategy to use joint ventures.

What Is a Joint Venture?

There is no easy answer to the question, "What is a joint venture?" Every institution or individual will have a different conception of what a joint venture is, because a joint venture is seldom regarded as an end in itself, but rather is viewed as a means of accomplishing a desired strategic, business, financial, or other objective. Nevertheless, it is helpful to define at least some of the major elements of a joint venture so that the efficacy of the joint venture strategy in a particular situation can be examined more objectively. Also, if the joint venture is pursued, the financial, legal, and medical aspects can then be focused upon clearly.

Almost any agreement or undertaking between a hospital and a physician or other organization can be described as a joint venture if it links the economic welfare of both parties. However, more precision is required in most business contexts because the establishment of a joint venture by a hospital with one or more physicians, with another hospital, or with another company will have many different implications.

To begin with, the characterization of a relationship between a hospital and a physician or physicians as a joint venture will have political consequences within the hospital's organizational structure and will have strategic consequences for the marketplace in which the hospital and the physicians operate. In effect, the characterization of the relationship as a joint venture will suggest to the nonparticipating physicians as well as to third parties that this hospital–physician relationship stands apart from the typical relationship that the physician or physicians have with the hospital as members of its active medical staff.

The characterization of a relationship between a hospital and its business partner as a joint venture also will have business implications. If a business transaction is characterized as a joint venture, it implies that the hospital and its business partner have at least partially integrated their businesses and have established common goals for the achievement of joint economic gain. This often means that one or both parties have given up exclusive control over the business or project that is the subject of the joint venture, and that some degree of economic interdependence has been created that involves the sharing of the opportunities for profit as well as the risks of loss.

From a legal standpoint, the characterization of a relationship between a hospital and its physician business partner will have significance in many different ways. The joint venture characterization of a relationship may have antitrust implications, may result in increased liability in one or more of the joint venturers, and may have significant federal or state income tax implications.

As can be seen from the foregoing discussion, the old saw, "When you've seen one joint venture, you've seen one joint venture!" may not be far off the mark. Joint ventures in ambulatory care typically will be dominated by the interests of hospitals and physicians. Therefore, most ambulatory joint ventures will have certain basic characteristics that will distinguish them from traditional hospital–medical staff relationships:

1. The joint venture typically will involve a legal relationship between a hospital and physicians that is separate and distinct from the medical staff–hospital relationship. Most often, these relationships will take the form of a separate contract, a separate partnership, or a separate corporation.

2. A joint venture will require the hospital and physicians to make an investment in a common enterprise that is distinct from and in addition to the hospital–medical staff relationship. This may be an investment of capital, services, technology, or some other asset.
3. A joint venture will require the sharing of control and risks in ways not previously common among hospitals and physicians. The degree to which control and risks are shared between the joint venturers will vary with the type of business and legal form selected.

As the preceding discussion suggests, a precise definition of a joint venture is not as important as clarity in the purposes and objectives of parties to the joint venture. Joint ventures may take a variety of forms, ranging from a simple contract to a business corporation with a complex capital structure. Each of the various possible forms will have its own legal, tax, and financial implications.

Contracts and Leases

A joint venture may consist of little more than a contract or lease between a hospital and a physician or physician group. The terms of the contract or lease might call for the hospital to provide the facilities (such as an ambulatory care center), equipment (such as an MRI scanner), and staff (such as technicians, nurses, and clerical personnel) for the venture, and call for the physicians to perform professional services. Properly drafted contracts and leases can result in the swift implementation of joint ventures that will further the various strategic and business objectives of the participants.

Partnerships and Corporations

In many cases, the terms of the joint venture will be more complex and will require the formation of a separate legal entity, such as a corporation or partnership. Numerous legal and tax considerations are involved in the selection of the corporate or partnership forms. In addition, there are numerous variations on the basic corporate and partnership forms, such as general partnerships, limited partnerships, regular corporations, closed corporations, and professional corporations. Moreover, there are different tax options available to corporations. Some corporations will be taxed as separate entities (C corporations) and others taxed in a manner similar to that of partnerships (S corporations).

Selection of Form

The form chosen for the venture should be the one that will best facilitate the achievement of the objectives of the hospital and physicians; in short, it should work for the venturers and not against them. The selection of the appropriate form for a joint venture will require consideration of a number of issues. The most important of these are:

- The degree to which some or all of the parties wish to either participate in or have no direct responsibility for the day-to-day management of the joint venture
- The tax objectives of the participants, usually taking into account the differences in tax objectives of taxable participants (such as individual physicians) and tax-exempt participants (such as not-for-profit, tax-exempt hospitals)
- The willingness of one or more parties to assume partial or complete responsibility for legal liabilities of the joint venture, including liability for the debts and obligations of the joint venture, its operating losses, and its professional liability

A Joint Venture as a New Strategic Relationship

It has been well documented in this book and elsewhere that changes in the delivery of ambulatory care are occurring at an unprecedented pace. These changes have stimulated various changes in the health care field that are having significant short- and long-term effects on hospitals and physicians and their relationships.

The financial, legal, political, and other changes have many direct effects upon hospitals and physicians, the primary providers of ambulatory care. First, hospitals are finding it increasingly necessary to restructure their existing ambulatory care programs to reduce costs, to make them more marketable, or to create appropriate utilization incentives. Similarly, hospitals without significant ambulatory care programs have, willingly or not, had to develop new programs to meet physician, consumer, or third-party payer demands. Finally, physicians have assumed a greater leadership role in the ambulatory care marketplace by increasingly attempting to garner additional market share with various forms of ambulatory care services.

The supply of new physicians, new entrepreneurial practice styles, and new hospital strategies will clearly result in winners and losers among hospitals, physicians, and medical groups. As a consequence, hospitals and physicians individually are seeking to optimize their own conditions through innovative practice opportunities, expansion, and vertical integration. Joint ventures increasingly are seen as providing a framework within which to modify individual goals for the sake of better overall performance.

Joint ventures are not, of course, the only means of achieving the various goals that hospitals and physicians seek. There clearly will remain numerous areas where the interests of hospitals and physicians will diverge and where it clearly will be advantageous for both players to maintain their independence. Nevertheless, there are increasing numbers of opportunities in which cooperation rather than conflict will be required.

Developing and Implementing Ambulatory Care Joint Ventures

As indicated at the outset, a joint venture should be viewed as a means of attaining business or strategic objectives, rather than as an end in and of itself. Consequently, the joint venture strategy must become part of the process of analyzing whether the institution will utilize a joint venture in connection with its service. Joint venture development as well as new business development frequently raises questions about the degree of risk the institution should undertake and the types of businesses to engage in.

Figure 3-2 depicts the joint venture development and implementation process. It begins, of course, with a clear definition of the services to be provided and the scope of the program to be joint ventured. It proceeds with various types of assessments to determine the feasibility of the joint venture as previously defined. During this assessment stage, it is common for the affected parties to make changes to the proposed service or program, cut back or expand service levels, and repeatedly test the financial and operational feasibility of the proposed business. During this stage, it is also important to reexamine periodically the issue of whether the joint venture is the appropriate means of achieving the strategic or business objectives. Failure to do so can result in the joint venture becoming the end rather than the means. This can be disastrous if developments during the feasibility process indicate that the use of a joint venture will not serve the originally intended purposes or could adversely affect the successful outcome of the project.

After these steps have been completed, the "go"–"no go" decision must be made at management and board levels. Unfortunately, because of securities law constraints and other legal limitations (for example, restrictions on the amount and percentage of money invested), it often is difficult for the hospital to obtain firm commitments from the physicians who potentially will become involved in the joint venture.

If a "go" decision is made, the process of implementation begins. This involves many concurrent tasks, such as the development of a more detailed business plan, the preparation of documents to make the offer, various presentations to physicians and the affected individuals, and the actual implementation of the development of the ambulatory care programs and facilities. After these tasks have been completed, the key ingredient to success will be proper execution of the business concept.

Overview of Legal Considerations for Joint Ventures

From legal and regulatory perspectives, joint ventures differ from many other types of health care ventures. The joining of hospitals and physicians in a single economic enterprise raises many new and complex legal and regulatory issues not applicable to separate ventures by hospitals or physicians.

Hospital–physician joint ventures are subject to several layers of law and regulation, from the federal level (federal tax and securities laws, the Medicare program's rules and regulations) to the state and local level (health planning and capital expenditure laws, licensing laws, and state Medicaid program

Figure 3-2. Joint Venture Development and Implementation Process

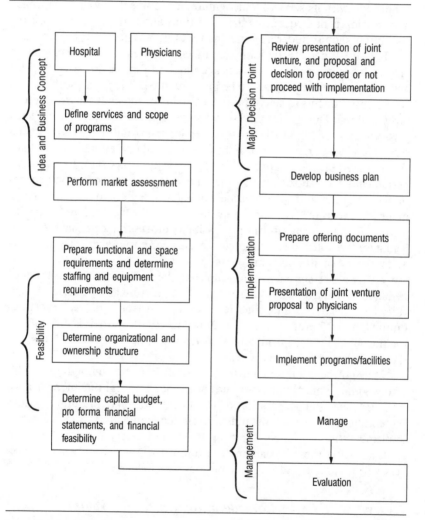

Source: Reprinted from *Joint Ventures between Hospitals and Physicians: A Competitive Strategy for the Healthcare Marketplace* by L. A. Burns and D. M. Mancino, pp. 33–34, with permission of Aspen Publishers, Inc., copyright 1987.

rules and regulations). These legal and regulatory provisions often overlap and occasionally conflict, adding to the complexities and uncertainties of establishing and operating ambulatory care joint ventures.

In addition, numerous forms of "private" regulation, such as the requirements of accreditation agencies and the requirements of insurance companies regarding coverage for services rendered to their insureds, can affect the structure, financing, and operations of joint ventures.

Put It in Writing

A discussion of all of the legal and regulatory issues that can affect joint ventures is beyond the scope of this chapter.[2] However, there are certain fundamental issues that should be addressed here regarding the legal documentation involved in the establishment of the joint venture itself.

The laws of the various states contain few statutory requirements applicable to joint ventures in general. For example, a general partnership can be formed with a handshake by the parties, and no written partnership agreement is even required. Although limited partnerships and corporations require the adoption and execution of limited partnership agreements or articles of incorporation and bylaws, all of which need to be in writing, the limited partnership and general business corporation laws of most states merely prescribe the minimum requirements to form these types of entities.

Although a handshake or oral "understanding" or "boilerplate" articles of incorporation and bylaws may be as legal and binding as comprehensive written agreements prepared by a capable attorney, they also may sow the seeds of discord between the parties and may eventually lead to expensive, destructive, and time-consuming lawsuits regarding the terms of the oral or incomplete agreement. The law reports are filled with cases involving litigation among partners and between shareholders and their corporations over unwritten terms and oral understandings.

For these reasons, it is essential that the parties to a joint venture negotiate and execute written agreements covering the significant business, economic, and tax aspects of the joint venture. Such written agreements should, at a minimum, address business and business opportunities, capital requirements, profits and losses, management, the timing of distributions, the maintenance of books and records, withdrawals and transfers, and termination.

The Business and Business Opportunities

The agreements should define the business of the joint venture and address whether similar or related business opportunities must be presented to the venturers for their consideration. The agreements should state how conflicts of interest regarding other business will be identified and resolved.

Capital Requirements

The agreements should identify the capital requirements of the joint venture and address such issues as the amount of capital to be contributed at the commencement of the joint venture, the amount of subsequent capital required to be contributed at later times during the life cycle of the joint venture, the manner in which further capital contributions may be compelled, and penalties for noncompliance with a capital call. Similar issues regarding indebtedness to be incurred during the term of the joint venture, both at its formation and in the future, should also be addressed.

Profits and Losses

One of the basic elements of any joint venture agreement will be the determination of each venturer's interest in the profits and losses of the business. Although general corporate law makes it easy to allocate profits and losses of a regular business corporation in accordance with share holdings, other joint venture forms, such as partnerships and closed corporations, will require careful attention to the issue of how profits and losses will be allocated.

Closely related to the issue of profits and losses are the factors that may be taken into account in determining profits and losses, such as whether or not profits attributable to appreciation in value of capital assets should be divided in the same proportion as profits from the operation of the joint venture.

Management

Issues concerning the management of the joint venture should be addressed. These issues will include: selection and removal of the board of directors of a corporate joint venture or the general partner or the management committee of a partnership joint venture; procedures to be followed to select and remove key management personnel; and methods to resolve deadlocks, particularly in those cases where the interests and voting power of the hospital and the physicians are equal. An example of this would be a prearranged commitment from an outside adviser, selected and agreed upon by both parties, to serve as an arbitrator.

The Timing of Distributions

The timing of distributions, such as dividends, should be addressed. When it comes to cash distributions, all venturers may not necessarily desire the same thing. The hospital general partner of a limited partnership, for example, may want the flexibility to withhold cash distributions to ensure that the partnership will always have sufficient funds on hand to cover its debts. On the other hand, physician limited partners may require that cash be distributed at specific times, thus reducing the amount of their investment at risk. It may also be appropriate to regulate cash distributions according to their sources, such as from normal operations, capital transactions, and refinancings.

The Maintenance of Books and Records

The joint venture documents should deal with such matters as bank accounts and investments and the authority of parties with regard to them. The documents should: require the maintenance of complete and accurate books of account and records relative to the joint venture business; specify the method of accounting to be used (for example, generally accepted accounting principles or a tax-based method of accounting); require interim and year-end financial reports and the preparation of federal, state, local, and other tax returns; and mandate the furnishing of relevant financial information to the joint venturers.

Withdrawals and Transfers

Provisions should be made for the withdrawals of venturers and for the transfers of interests in the venture. Even if transfers of interests are generally prohibited, certain types of transfers are inevitable. Examples of these are transfers that will occur by law upon death or typically will be compelled by the venture documents as a result of such occurrences as loss of license, medical staff privileges, or malpractice insurance; disability of one of the individual joint venturers; or acquisition of interest in a competing enterprise.

Termination

Appropriate provision should be made for the termination of the joint venture and for the division and distribution of its assets upon dissolution. In this regard, the documents may include rights of first refusal to purchase fixed assets and other tangible and intangible property of the joint venture, and provisions regarding control over such business records as patient records, client lists, and other proprietary information.

Tax Planning for Joint Ventures

Physicians and hospitals willing to commit risk capital in joint ventures are entitled to a number of tax benefits, including the immediate deduction of certain costs normally encountered during initial start-up and capitalization and the rapid recovery of other costs. The primary tax objective in planning and implementing a joint venture will be the maximization of such benefits, thus reducing the total tax bill payable by the joint venture and its owners. However, planning to accomplish this objective must be considered within the context of the business objectives of the venturers because at some point the accomplishment of business planning objectives may outweigh the total maximization of any tax benefits involved.

If a joint venture and its participants are to maximize the tax benefits available to them, at least three results should be achieved. First, the tax economics of the joint venture should result in the deferral of the payment of taxes that would otherwise be due currently. This can be accomplished in a number of ways, such as by maximizing the accelerated cost recovery deductions available to the venture.[3] Second, tax planning by tax-exempt hospitals and related tax-exempt organizations may result, if properly structured, in the realization of income that is totally exempt from taxation. Third, tax-exempt hospitals and their tax-exempt affiliates must structure their direct or indirect participation in a joint venture in a manner that will avoid jeopardizing their tax-exempt status.[4]

Fraud and Abuse Aspects of Joint Ventures

Joint venture participants must be extremely sensitive to the potential application of federal and state laws that seek to prohibit such abusive practices as kickbacks and other payments made or offered to induce or in exchange for patient referrals. These laws, which often have criminal and civil penalties for their violation, may apply to hospitals and their affiliates, freestanding facilities, physicians and other professionals, and a new entity created to serve as the vehicle through which the ambulatory care joint venture will be conducted. In addition, the U.S. Congress has recently extended the civil enforcement authority of the inspector general of the Department of Health and Human Services by providing for significant civil sanctions, such as termination of provider status, in the event that improper conduct is found to exist.

Compliance with both federal and state fraud and abuse laws is made difficult by the realities of the competitive environment in which most hospitals and physicians function today. First, most ambulatory care joint ventures are volume sensitive. Thus, such joint ventures require certain levels of patient referrals or utilization in order to break even or to achieve projected levels of profitability. However, no matter how tempting an arrangement may be in terms of ensuring the referrals or utilization necessary to maintain financial viability, any arrangement that presents a substantial risk of violating a federal or state criminal statute should be avoided. Second, the extremely competitive environment in ambulatory care rewards those hospitals and physicians for moving swiftly and decisively to initiate a new service and gain market share. The tension between complying with the law and competing effectively is heightened because federal and state fraud and abuse statutes often are vague, and although there has been considerable enforcement activity, such activity has not resulted in a meaningful number of cases and rulings that can serve as precedents. Moreover, safe harbor regulations provide little comfort for most joint ventures.

Where possible, joint venture participants should obtain advance opinions from government officials with respect to the propriety of entering into a joint venture. In addition, opinions of counsel, valuations of equipment, evaluations of lease terms and financing arrangements, and similar strategies will be helpful in reducing the risk that any particular form of joint venture will be found at a later date to be in violation of federal or state fraud and abuse laws.

Finally, participants should monitor federal and state legislative initiatives that may limit or preclude physician ownership of health providers to which those physicians refer patients.

Joint Ventures as a Strategy

Joint ventures will continue to serve as vehicles for hospitals and others to restructure existing ambulatory care programs and to develop new ones. They make hospitals, physicians, and others more economically interdependent by, among other things, enabling all parties to participate in the rewards and risks of a successful or unsuccessful ambulatory care business venture.

One of the keys to the success of joint ventures, in addition to mutual commitment of time, capital, and professional expertise, is a recognition of the need for different types of managerial talent. In addition, all levels of an existing hospital organization, as well as the physicians and managers of the new venture, are likely to require skills different from those that they typically utilize today. Some of the important factors that determine the success or failure of the joint ventures are the type of planning that has been undertaken, the type of legal structure that is utilized, and the type of financial resources that are committed to the joint venture. However, one of the most important factors is the actual ability of the joint venture, once it has been established, to develop and package its products and services effectively to meet its competition and to maintain and increase its market share and profitability.

The trend toward the use of joint ventures will continue to result in the differentiation of hospitals by their clinical product lines and services, legal and financial structures utilized to deliver those services, and the nature of their returns on their investments in such services. Joint ventures in ambulatory care are not merely a passing fancy, but are a viable strategic option for dealing with professional, economic, and community responsibilities.

Conclusion

The laws and regulations that affect aggressive development of ambulatory care services often create a complicated maze through which hospitals and other participants must navigate carefully. This task is made difficult by the many layers and inconsistencies of the laws and regulations affecting ambulatory care programs. In some cases, incentives are provided for establishing ambulatory care programs as freestanding entities, but other legal requirements may adversely affect the ability of such freestanding ambulatory care programs to operate efficiently. Further complexities are added by the formal and informal practices of private regulators, such as accreditation agencies, insurance companies, and lenders.

This chapter has considered only a few of the numerous legal and regulatory issues affecting hospitals that wish to expand existing or develop new ambulatory care programs independently or through joint ventures. Good legal planning facilitates good business planning, because the timely identification of legal or structural issues can minimize start-up or development costs and maximize operational efficiencies.

References

1. Burns, L. A., and Mancino, D. M. *Joint Ventures between Hospitals and Physicians: A Competitive Strategy for the Healthcare Marketplace.* Rockville, MD: Aspen Publishers, Inc., 1987.

2. Burns and Mancino.

3. Stromberg, R., and Bowman, C. *Joint Ventures for Hospitals and Physicians: Legal Considerations.* Chicago: American Hospital Publishing, Inc., 1986.

4. Stromberg and Bowman.

Chapter 4

Examining the Options in Facilities Planning

Thomas P. Berry and Alice D'Alessio

To reorganize services for enhanced ambulatory care, the hospital should explore both the functional and the facility options open to it. From a functional standpoint, a number of possibilities exist. A hospital can probably establish a small, independent, on-campus ambulatory care service area in its present facilities. It can also establish off-campus satellites for primary and urgent care that would act as referral centers for the hospital. It can create freestanding or off-campus entrepreneurial centers, perhaps in joint ventures with physicians. These freestanding centers can include magnetic resonance imaging facilities, multimodality and diagnostic centers, surgery centers, and cancer treatment buildings.

The hospital may wish to convert part of its medical office space into a group practice center, joining independent physicians together under hospital sponsorship (see chapter 5). The hospital can establish new, campus-based primary care or multispecialty group practice centers. Another possibility is forming campus-based centers of excellence that integrate, for example, a cardiology group with a hospital-based cardiac care and rehabilitation program. This approach involves unbundling the outpatient services of the hospital and forming new combinations of outpatient and inpatient services that make the most sense.

A number of facility options also exist. The hospital can renovate existing hospital or medical office space for ambulatory care, or it can build new facilities on or off campus. An analysis of the hospital's specific market by means of a marketing and business plan enables the hospital to determine which is the most appropriate decision.

Obviously, the function of the facility is the first consideration. At one end of the scale is a small renovation of an existing clinic to facilitate expanded ambulatory care services; at the other end is an all-new, comprehensive ambulatory care center to accommodate a complete unbundling and regrouping of hospital services.

With the new outpatient mind-set, the hospital should look at what services it offers now, decide what it wants to become, and establish a plan for getting there. The typical present hospital facility has inpatient beds. It has intensive and cardiac care units, surgical and recovery areas, rehabilitation facilities of all sorts, diagnostic services, and therapy departments such as oncology, radiation oncology, and physical therapy. It has central stores and supplies and perhaps programs geared toward health promotion and wellness.

All these activities need to be analyzed in terms of intensity and function. Then the outpatient and inpatient activities should be separated so that the high-cost, intensive inpatient services—inpatient beds, intensive care, and surgery—are used primarily for inpatients and are located close to one another. Outpatient activities, such as rehabilitation, diagnostic services, therapy, storage and distribution, administration, and physician services to outpatients, can be in another area or building that has a new look and a different atmosphere.

A Blueprint for Action

In forming a blueprint for action for increased ambulatory care, the first question that arises is whether to remodel or build a new facility. This is a difficult area in which to offer advice, because every situation is different and few "wide brush" rules apply.

Remodeling an Existing Building

One of the main reasons for a hospital to consider remodeling is that if it does not, several staff or board members are bound to ask why this option was not considered. Remodeling has certain undeniable advantages. Obviously, the new services will be in close proximity to the present facility and programs. They will be in an existing building on an existing site, so the hospital does not need to find or commit additional land. If the area to be remodeled is separated functionally from the main operation, the remodeling can perhaps proceed with a minimum of disruption to the rest of the facility. Remodeling is often seen as cheaper than building new space. However, the cost of remodeling can easily approach or exceed the cost of new facilities. One reason is that work in an existing building can often trigger building code retrofits.

Existing structural patterns may not be appropriate for outpatient use. For example, a typical hospital bay (space between columns) is 24 feet wide. Typical outpatient spacing varies widely, but the most common bay is often

28 feet. Added to that may be a 12-foot procedure room in the middle, and another corridor at 4 feet, making a bay of 44 feet. Finally, if a deep suite and another row of examination rooms at the back of the procedure rooms is desired, the bay would need to be 56 feet. These bays, 28, 44, and 56 feet, are the most popular and flexible bay sizes for outpatient facilities. They have been used over and over again primarily because they work. Unfortunately, hospital-based column spacing does not match these dimensions, which means that a column could end up in the middle of a room or that rooms must be bigger and less efficient.

The shape of the hospital may not be correct for outpatient facilities. A number of hospitals are long and narrow, with double-loaded corridors, consisting of a single corridor down the center of the building. Outpatient space should be concentrated in a block shape for more efficiency. An area that is too large will end up having too many interior spaces with no windows.

Mechanical systems frequently need extensive retrofits for outpatient use. Most space that is going to be renovated is old, which means that the systems may have reached the end of their life. Also, heating systems were originally designed to serve one patient in a hospital room rather than one or two patients and a physician in smaller examination rooms as well as waiting rooms with more people and activity. The space will probably have to be air-conditioned all year long because of the increased heat load.

Another consideration is the atmosphere of the space. Hospital space may not lend itself to creating the kind of welcoming, comfortable ambience that is so important when trying to attract outpatients. Segregating inpatients and outpatients within the existing facility may also be difficult. All of these factors must be taken into account when analyzing the potential for remodeling. Existing space may seem attractive, but the compromises necessary to make it into an effective outpatient facility often tip the scales toward new construction.

Selecting a Site for a New Building

Finding and selecting the proper site for a new building must proceed in an orderly way. Realtors can provide a book of available real estate, but because they probably do not understand the health care business, their advice may not be useful. Frequently the committee established for overseeing a new facility appoints a subcommittee that includes people who know the town and understand what land is worth. The committee should include a professional, such as the architect–engineer, construction manager, or designer–builder, who can provide cost estimates to show what each site would cost to develop as well as assess which sites present the most attractive possibilities from a nonfinancial point of view.

The criteria for site selection should be set by the building committee, and top priorities should be determined before the committee goes to look at land. Doing so will prevent committee members from making judgments based on preconceived ideas. Setting the criteria can be complex, but useful guidelines are available, such as *Site Selection for Health Care Facilities,* by James Lifton and Owen B. Hardy.[1] The book itemizes criteria to be used when determining an appropriate site for either a hospital or an outpatient facility. In terms of outpatient facilities, the two main areas to be considered are financial, or objective, factors and nonfinancial, or subjective, factors.

Financial Factors

The costs of site acquisition and site preparation are two financial factors that must be considered. Acquisition costs include the base purchase price, plus the cost of any options necessary to purchase additional land to make the site usable, plus the cost of that additional land, minus any anticipated proceeds from sell-offs of unneeded land.

Preparation costs include demolition of unusable existing buildings, if any; utilities such as electricity, gas and fuel, water, and sewer; grading and filling the site to create a platform on which to build; and providing drainage and protection from groundwater. Any footing and foundation costs over and above normal construction and any miscellaneous preparation costs are also in this category.

Nonfinancial Factors

A scoring system for nonfinancial factors is very subjective and complex, but establishing the priorities early can help to prevent conflict later in the selection process. A suggested maximum score for each item in the following scoring system appears in parentheses:

1. Proximity to patients (12)
2. Adequate size of usable area—allows for future expansion (11)
3. Major road visibility and access (10)
4. Proximity to personal services, such as shopping centers, banks, and so forth (10)
5. Favorable configuration and orientation, including slope, prevailing winds, and so forth (8)
6. Proximity to other health care facilities, especially hospitals (8)
7. Lack of easements and restrictions (7)
8. Direct access (7)
9. Favorable zoning aspects (outpatient center can be built under existing zoning; requirements for area, height, and parking are acceptable; surrounding land use is acceptable) (6)
10. Accessibility to city services and utilities (5)

11. Neighborhood amenities—views, noise, odor, and so forth (10)
12. No negative environmental impact (3)
13. Long-term desirability (10)
14. Short-term desirability (10)[2]

To illustrate this concept, any score above 81 would indicate an excellent site. A score of 61 to 80 would indicate a good site; from 41 to 60, a fair site; and below 40, a poor site. Using the nonfinancial scores alone would enable the hospital to select an excellent site but one that may not leave enough budget to build the building. Obviously, the scores must be combined with the financial data in some meaningful way. Three simple methods are suggested in the Lifton-Hardy booklet, and a fourth is a hybrid of the others.

- *Set the budget for site acquisition and choose the best site within the budget.* This method may be too inflexible and demands some realistic site development costs. The danger is that an otherwise excellent site may be disqualified on cost alone.
- *Set the lowest acceptable score for the nonfinancial aspects and choose the least expensive site that meets that score.* Again, this method could result in choosing a site that is only marginally acceptable and missing a far better site at only a slightly higher cost.
- *Pick an overall value for each site by dividing the site cost by the nonfinancial score to get the cost-of-quality ratio, or the dollar-for-quality point.* For example, if a site costs $2 million and has a score of 75 points, each point is worth $26,666. This method gives a better notion of the trade-off between cost and quality. However, problems exist at the ends of the spectrum. For instance, a high value per point may be too low on overall quality for the project. In other words, low cost and low quality could produce a high ratio.
- *Use a hybrid method that allows you to decide the same way you shop for any product or service.* Set the maximum cost to be paid and the minimum level of acceptable quality and pick the best value that meets both criteria.

Space Programming

Space programming is the process by which the building committee can determine how much space is required in the facility to fulfill the business plan. In the simplest terms, it involves asking all the persons involved what they want and need in the new space and recording it in a matrix format that is usable for the design team. The program must be used as a yardstick for all later work. If properly done, this assessment can tell users a lot about what the facility needs in order to operate.

The first step in the program is to set guidelines from which project members can program the space they need. If you do not set up guidelines, some participants in the project may demand a room that is considerably larger than the rest, and complain that their requirements were not considered when they do not get what they asked for. Setting standard guidelines enables you to stay ahead of the people being interviewed.

The next thing to decide is exactly how the facility is going to function in terms of examination rooms and consultation rooms. A couple of standard room organizations are frequently used in outpatient care. The first is what many people call the "Mayo" plan, which combines examination space with office and consultation space in a single room. This arrangement does not allow high volume, because the physician normally leaves the room while the patient changes clothes, which cuts down on efficient movement and use of time.

The second concept is one of individual turf, or the idea that a physician's rooms are his or hers alone. When that physician is not on the premises, however, the space goes to waste.

A more efficient approach is what is known as flex space, where a series of examination rooms are shared. Physicians each have their own consultation room but then use differing combinations of the same examination rooms, depending on their own scheduling. The advantage to flex space is maximum utilization of space. One disadvantage is that the only turf physicians have are their own offices.

When setting the dimensions for room size, the planner should insist, if possible, that all consultation and examination rooms be the same size so that they can be switched from one use to another with a minimum of rearranging. The main goal of the programming effort is to ensure that all rooms are in use as much of the time as possible in order to control fixed costs. With the dimensions established and graphically represented, the planner should arrange a series of meetings with department chiefs, who provide the space "wish list" for each department. This "wish list" provides the necessary general information about each department: the number of full-time equivalents or physicians who are available at any one time; the number of staff members; the current and prospective levels of encounters; the hours and days of operation; and a list of which departments need to be near or prefer not to be near which other departments.

Next, the planner prepares a room-by-room listing of exactly what each department needs, being careful to determine who is working in each room and when, in order to identify as much as possible any special equipment needs. Spaces that can be shared with others need to be identified, as do spaces that cannot be shared. For example, surgical and gastrointestinal departments do not share space well because surgery cases usually require minimal cleanup, whereas gastrointestinal procedures may require extensive cleanup after procedures are performed.

When all the department spaces have been ascertained, the planner tallies them and adds them together to determine the total space of the facility. The planner reviews this space with the administration and compares it with the business plan. If necessary, the planner may have to return to various departments and reprogram their areas until the total space is in compliance with the business plan. At this point, the planner may want to suggest that two physicians or two departments share the same space to reduce the area of the program. The planner will also want to verify with departments that proposed patient volume levels justify the space requested.

To the total department space, the planner adds 20 to 30 percent for departmental circulation, and another 20 to 30 percent for building circulation. In states with strict handicap codes, the planner must add the larger figure to comply with these requirements. The total figure tells how many square feet the new facility has to have. Because outpatient spaces tend to be smaller and more efficient, what appears to be a tight space program by inpatient standards may be optimal for outpatient care. One rule of thumb for outpatient care that often applies is to provide 1,200 to 1,500 square feet per full-time equivalent provider.

Figure 4-1 shows how space was used within 18 different clinics. Only 20 to 25 percent of the space in these facilities actually generates income. The rest is support space.

Determining Specific Project Cost

Determining specific project cost is a crucial step in the planning process. Once the total area has been decided, the planner can arrive at a cost per square foot of the facility. However, cost per square foot is a calculation that has a number of different meanings, depending on what is included and what method is used to measure it. The American Institute of Architects and the Building Owners Maintenance Association (BOMA) each use different methods of area calculations, and many estimators have worked out their own way of calculating area. The choice of a calculation method directly affects cost. For example, one person may measure a building at 54,000 square feet, and another may measure the same building at 55,000 square feet. If the total cost is the same, the cost of the square foot per building is not.

When comparing costs per square foot, the planner must be sure that the spaces are being tabulated consistently and must have a clear understanding of what is included in the cost. One definition that is preferred includes everything that the project team is controlling: building structure, finishes, wall treatments, cabinetry, and HVAC (heating, ventilating, and air-conditioning), as well as architectural and engineering fees and any construction management fees. Not included in this figure are medical equipment, furniture, artwork, or any site-development costs. In this way, the cost per square foot of an outpatient building can be fairly easily compared

Figure 4-1.   Clinic Space Usage

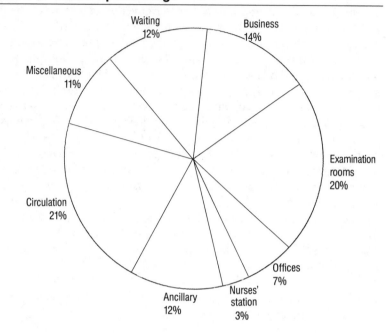

Source: Marshall Erdman and Associates, Madison, Wisconsin, 1989.

among different buildings as well as between the different delivery options of construction management versus design–build because all categories except those specifically listed.are included. Construction management refers to the joint responsibility of construction and of the architectural firm to oversee design and construction, whereas design–build means that a single firm has responsibility for all construction and architectural decisions.

For the purposes of our discussion, assume that a typical outpatient building with physicians' offices will cost about $85 per square foot in the middle of the country, $105 on the West Coast, $70 in the Deep South, and perhaps $95 in the Northeast. This spread from $70 to $105 points out one of the problems with cost per square foot. These cost projections are from 1987, and the project cost time frames that they apply to are based on a design–build schedule rather than on a traditional architect draw–bid–build schedule, where the architectural firm serves as the sole agent of the hospital with total responsibility for project completion. Of the various methods available to the hospital, the design–build schedule tends to involve the shortest amount of time between conception of the project and completion.

The most important influence on the cost per square foot is the mix of function in the planned facility. The formula is dynamic and can change radically, with, for instance, the addition of a surgery room or special shielding for magnetic resonance imaging. Care and professional assistance is needed to avoid problems with cost per square foot.

The following examples illustrate a range of costs and development time for a number of facility options. All costs were based in Madison, Wisconsin, in 1987.

Freestanding Primary Care Center

In its simplest form, the freestanding primary care center is a doctor's office for family practice, which is the gatekeeper function of medicine. It can be any size but most often is somewhere around 2,500 square feet. This kind of building requires a site of ¼ to ½ acre to accommodate the building, parking, circulation, and green space. Figure 4-2 shows the program for a freestanding primary care center, as well as the spatial relationships. Ideal circulation in this particular building will get people into the inner space and a treatment room or examination room quickly. Once the patient is in a room, the assistant can go back to the reception desk or to the nurses' station. The concept here is to move the staff, not the patient, because moving the patient uses up a staff member. Fewer staff members may be needed if they are not required to move patients, thereby reducing salary and benefit expenses. Patients are not allowed to penetrate too far into the suite, and the nurses' station is located centrally so that nurses can watch all of the rooms and be close to the action.

Figure 4-2. Freestanding Primary Care Center (2,600 square feet)

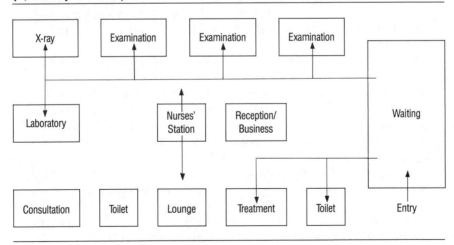

Source: Marshall Erdman and Associates, Madison, Wisconsin, 1989.

Examination rooms are clustered, enabling a physician to go easily from one to the next. The patient can stop at the reception desk or business office on the way out to pay the bill without having to stand in the waiting room. In this particular concept, consultation can be done in the examination room as well as in a specially designated room.

Having a staff lounge is important even though the building is small. Staff members still need a place to "get away." The small laboratory and X-ray room are located to the rear, because not every patient needs to go in one or the other of those rooms. Specimens can be gathered in the rest-room just off the nurses' station. A building such as this can be built for somewhere between $80 and $85 per square foot and takes approximately two months in design, two months in working drawings, and five months for construction.

Freestanding Ambulatory Surgery Center

A four- or six-operating-room (OR) freestanding ambulatory surgery center can be accommodated in approximately 13,000 square feet of floor area, as shown in figure 4-3. A freestanding building this size requires approximately 1¼ to 1½ acres for parking, green space, and setbacks. The spatial relationships of this building are completely different from the primary care center because of the different traffic patterns required by functions performed in the building.

The patient flow is circular, with patients entering the flow at the reception room and waiting room to check in. People who have accompanied the patient wait here or are told to return. The patient leaves the reception area, goes into the preoperative area, disrobes, and either gets onto a gurney or sits in an easy chair. Some centers have chairs for the patient to sit in while an intravenous infusion is started, but many others have the patients on gurneys even if they are ambulatory. This way patient movement can be controlled.

Clothing can be taken care of in a number of ways. It can be placed in a sterile bag attached to the gurney. It can also be placed in a locker that opens from the preoperative side as well as from the secondary recovery side. These double-faced lockers enable patients to get their clothes from the other side after the procedure. Many centers use a locker area that is connected to both preoperative and recovery rooms so that nurses can pick up the clothing for patients once they have recovered.

Programming for the preoperative area can be complex. As procedures become more invasive, more work is done on the patients in the preoperative area before they go into the ORs. Some centers like to use a pre-preoperative room for complicated cases so that they are able to complete the preoperative procedures on one patient while the previous patient is finishing up in the OR next door. This setup maximizes the doctor's turnaround time, but this

Figure 4-3. Freestanding Six-Operating-Room Ambulatory Surgery Center (13,000 square feet)

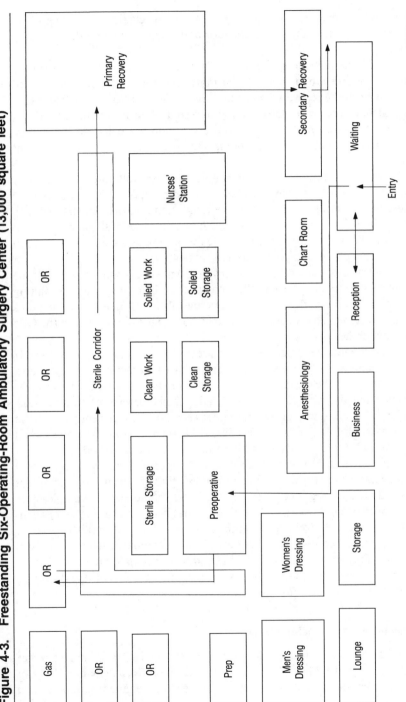

Source: Marshall Erdman and Associates, Madison, Wisconsin, 1989.

approach is obviously not appropriate for all specialties. The patient then walks or rides into the sterile corridor and finally right into the operating room.

After the procedure, the patient is wheeled into the primary recovery area. Here beds are separated by curtains. The nurses' station is positioned so that both the recovery rooms and the sterile corridor are visible. Many centers have a separate glassed-in room to control the noise level for difficult recoveries or for children. Each recovery station normally has full oxygen and suction capabilities. The rooms should be as bright and cheerful as possible.

When patients are awake and stable, they can walk into the secondary recovery area, where there are chairs instead of beds. This area should be close to the waiting room so that the family can join the patients and help them dress. Having a nurses' station here is also helpful for patient and family. The patient then dresses and leaves by a separate door, not through the waiting room and past incoming patients.

The flow of personnel in this arrangement is different from that in the primary care center. An anesthesiology office is located near the waiting room so that the patient can come in a day ahead of time for instructions. This location makes it easy for the anesthesiologist to go between the ORs and his or her office.

A side entrance somewhere near the dressing area should be used by staff to enter and leave the center. Many centers have separate staff and physician dressing areas. The preference, however, is for male and female dressing areas that are shared by physicians and staff, rather than four separate dressing areas. A room for soiled instruments and linens should be conveniently located so that materials follow a fairly direct dirty–clean–sterile path. The center should always have more storage space than was originally estimated.

The environment in a surgery center is crucial. Sensitivity to patients means not having the recovering patient exit through the waiting room, but instead having a separate covered exit. Colors should be light and pleasant, and rooms should have a high level of natural light. Above all, the inpatient mind-set must be avoided, because such a mind-set will result in a larger facility than necessary at higher cost. A fairly compact surgery center can be built for somewhere between $105 and $110 per square foot. It will take approximately three months in design, three months in working drawings, and six months for construction.

Diagnostic and Imaging Center

With the exception of magnetic resonance, the diagnostic and imaging center shown in figure 4-4 has all ancillary services presently in demand. They can be accommodated in about 11,000 square feet and require between 1¼ and 1½ acres.

Figure 4-4. Diagnostic and Imaging Center (11,000 square feet)

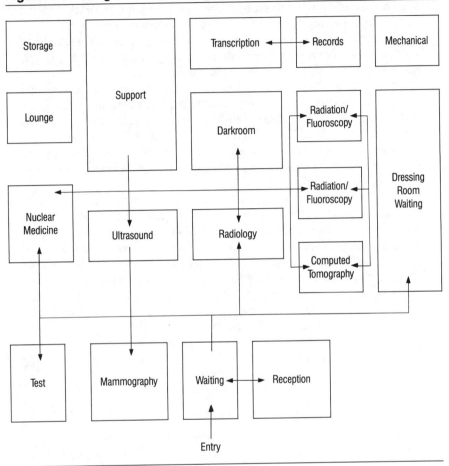

Source: Marshall Erdman and Associates, Madison, Wisconsin, 1989.

The spatial relationships shown in figure 4-4 are particular to imaging centers. For highest efficiency, the patient and the staff should have separate circulation paths. Patients follow a direct path. They enter at the front door, check in at the counter, and wait for their procedure. They are escorted into a dressing area, helped to disrobe as necessary, gowned, and then either directed to wait in a preprocedure waiting area or in the dressing room, if it is large enough. If preprocedure areas are used, male and female patients should be separated. Dressing rooms should be large enough and bright enough that the patient does not feel claustrophobic.

A technical assistant takes the patient from the waiting room, preprocedure room, or dressing room into the imaging room for the procedure. The patient is then escorted back to the dressing room or to a bathroom adjacent to the radiation/fluoroscopy room that then connects back into the hallway and dressing room. The patient then dresses and leaves.

Staff circulation is on the other side of the imaging rooms. Patient and staff paths do not cross until they meet in the imaging room. This arrangement makes staff movement very efficient.

The darkroom is centrally located for easy accessibility by staff for film delivery and pickup. A transcription station is located away from the patient paths and adjacent to medical records. A staff support room is behind the patient areas to allow for free movement without patient interaction.

Mammography is done in a separate area that has its own dressing and waiting area. Interior finishes, art, and lighting should project warmth, comfort, and reassurance.

The planners of a diagnostic facility must remember that it needs to accommodate only outpatients, not patients on gurneys who need complex procedures. The facility should be lean and mean in space usage, because the equipment and building portion takes large amounts of space, and is always there, whether 10 or 50 scans a day are being done. Therefore, all peripheral space should be kept to an absolute minimum.

A diagnostic center generally costs between $95 and $100 per square foot. This cost does not include magnetic resonance imaging but does include a CT scanner. Also not included are the costs for the equipment, processors and special equipment, or shielding. Buildings such as this can be designed in three to four months, take another three months in working drawings, and take six months for construction.

Magnetic Resonance Imaging Center

A magnetic resonance imaging center accommodating a single 1.5 Tesla magnet to operate the imagers requires 3,000 to 4,000 square feet and requires approximately ½ acre of land (figure 4-5). The single function of the building is to support an expensive piece of imaging equipment. Families of patients may be in the building for a fairly long time and may require adequate waiting space.

Once again, a proper traffic flow helps keep staff at a minimum. Patients enter, check in at the reception counter, and sit down to wait for their examination. The receptionist should lock up jewelry or other metallic objects and valuables at the desk, because magnets can destroy credit cards and stop watches. For peace of mind, patients with pacemakers can be issued a nonmetallic key to their storage drawer.

The receptionist escorts patients to the dressing room, where they disrobe and perhaps put on a gown. Patients then wait in a waiting room or preprocedure room that should have access to a toilet. The receptionist returns to the desk to control the front of the building. The technician then

Figure 4-5. Magnetic Resonance Imaging Center (3,724 square feet)

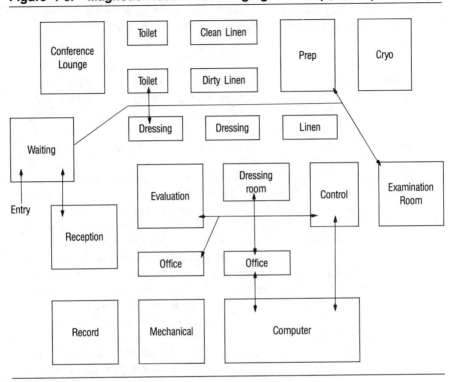

Source: Marshall Erdman and Associates, Madison, Wisconsin, 1989.

escorts previous patients off the couch and into their dressing rooms and takes waiting patients into the examination room. Previous patients then dress and proceed to the front desk.

A preparation room is often being used now for prescan procedures, particularly if an infusion is called for. The preparation room can also accommodate wheelchair or stretcher patients from nearby hospitals, who are brought in through a separate entrance and are shielded from the waiting room but are within sight of the reception desk.

The staff functions in a tight circle to minimize distance. Their path goes from the control room to the dressing room to the examination room to the control room and perhaps to the computer room. Physicians can stay in the evaluation room–control room–darkroom circle. The technologist's room should be right in the center for easy access to equipment.

A building housing a magnetic resonance imager (MRI) can probably be built for $150 per square foot. That cost would include the cost of the building as well as the radio frequency shielding and special mechanical-electrical equipment required by the magnet. It would not include, however, the cost of a power conditioner. Such MRI projects typically come together very quickly. They can take approximately two months in design, one to two months in working drawings, and five months to complete the project.

Cancer Treatment Center

The cancer treatment center shown in figure 4-6 has two linear accelerators, one simulator, and associated support spaces, all in approximately 5,800 square feet. This building would require between ½ and ¾ of an acre of land for parking and setbacks. Accelerator buildings serve two distinct groups of patients. One group is new to the procedure. These patients come for an examination and work-up of molds and simulation. The other group consists of patients who return on a regular basis to receive their treatment.

New patients check in at the reception window, go to the dressing room at the top of the plan, disrobe as necessary, go into the simulator room for work-up, return to the dressing room, dress, and leave. Perhaps the process will include a consultation, an examination, or patient education.

Returning patients arrive, check in, and go to the dressing area where they are gowned, if necessary. They wait in the sub-waiting area for their procedure. Patients go into the accelerator room, receive their treatment, and then return to the dressing area, dress, and leave. The procedure, including the necessary setup time, is time-consuming, and volume is not as high as in other facilities.

The staff functions in two sections, as in an MRI facility. Technicians are in the back section, running the procedure or helping in the simulator. The receptionist or business agent is in front of the building controlling that portion, and the physician and physicist are in the staff area for consultation and treatment planning.

A key point to remember about a cancer treatment center is that many of the patients are very ill and may even be terminal. The environment should be as pleasant as possible. At all costs, this kind of center should not be in a basement devoid of natural light. Many centers use skylights in waiting areas and preprocedure areas and sometimes even in procedure rooms, depending on what equipment and shielding are necessary. To deemphasize the serious nature of the equipment, the designer should be particularly mindful of color, art, and other humanizing detail.

A cancer treatment facility normally costs around $150 per square foot and can be designed in two to three months, drawn in two months, and built in six to seven months.

Multispecialty Group Practice Center

Figure 4-7 shows a multispecialty group practice facility of approximately 50,000 square feet. Such a center requires somewhere between 5 and 6 acres of land, including land for on-grade parking.

Figure 4-6. Cancer Treatment Center—Double-Accelerator Facility (5,840 square feet)

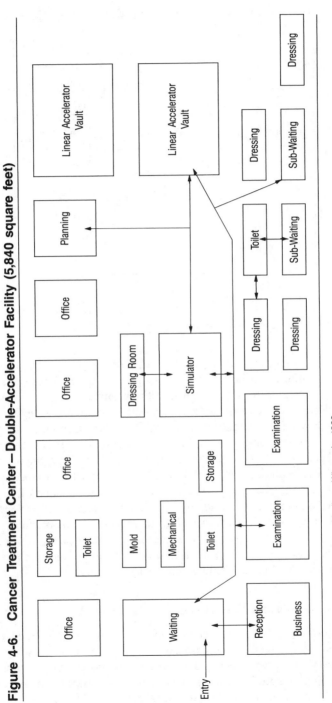

Source: Marshall Erdman and Associates, Madison, Wisconsin, 1989.

Figure 4-7.   Multispecialty Group Practice Center (50,000 square feet)

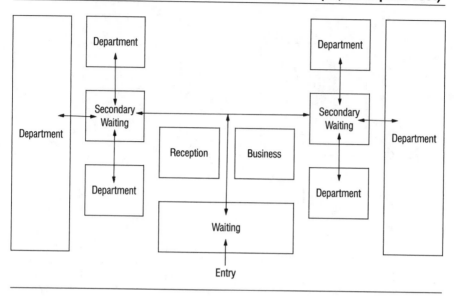

Source: Marshall Erdman and Associates, Madison, Wisconsin, 1989.

Entering patients should check in at an entrance counter, then go to a secondary waiting area near the department they are visiting. The person who accompanied them to the clinic stays in a waiting room close to the door. Patient traffic radiates outward from the secondary waiting rooms and reception area. Doctors and staff circulate through the waiting rooms without crossing the patients coming or going. Business functions are concentrated at the entrance to help the patient on either the way in or the way out. Departments allow free ebb and flow into each other as the caseload changes. For instance, clinics may rotate. Orthopedics may be on Monday afternoons, but not on Tuesdays, when rheumatology meets and uses those same examination rooms. A 50,000-square-foot multispecialty care group practice facility probably costs somewhere between $85 and $90 per square foot. It can be designed in three to four months, drawn in three months, built in an additional nine months, and can be hospital-based or freestanding from a hospital.

Integrated Ambulatory Care Center

The hospital-based or freestanding integrated ambulatory care center represents a multidimensional approach to the delivery of ambulatory care. Generally, this facility represents the *center for excellence approach,* which combines hospital outpatient departments with specifically related physicians' offices in what would ordinarily be a medical office building. These buildings can range in size from 5,000 to 6,000 square feet to well over 100,000 square feet. Because of the complexity of developing an integrated ambulatory care center, a complete discussion is in chapter 5, "Integrating Ambulatory Care Expansion with Physicians' Offices."

Reviewing the Planning Concepts

In summary, some key planning concepts are common to any type of center:

- Separation of staff and patient movement is important for efficiency and economy. In an outpatient facility, everyone is moving. Traffic patterns require particular attention:
  - Patients should be kept as close as possible to the waiting room. Their movement should be controlled, and the path between waiting room and examination room should be kept simple and short so that patients can find their way easily.
  - The distance that staff has to travel should be kept to a minimum.
- Areas for the greeting and check-in functions and the reappointment and payment functions should be separate so that patients are not required to stand in the middle of the waiting room while they schedule their next procedure or talk about their bill.
- Room sizes should be consistent in order to have maximum flexibility of use and ease of remodeling.
- The facility should be able to accommodate expansion easily without compromising the planning doctrine.

The Feasibility Study

In order to study the options and facility plans in detail, the project team should prepare a feasibility study. A feasibility study tells the building committee or board how big the facility should be; where the facility should be; how, when, and why the facility should be built; and how much it will cost. If any of these elements are left out, decision makers may not be willing to make the decision to proceed.

The feasibility study should include:

1. A statement setting out the ground rules and parameters and the program that has resulted from interviews and tabulations. All details should be put in the summary at the front of the study. This program becomes the space yardstick for future design work so that the design team is always designing the same amount of building as was called for in the program.
2. Block diagrams that show how the departments will be arranged within the building, who is going to be near whom, and how they will relate to the multistory structure.

3. A site analysis and usage that shows the building footprint with parking and site utilization, including site-selection criteria.
4. A projected cost model that is as detailed as possible. Blanks will serve as reminders for future work and research. All the assumptions that were used to develop the cost model should be included, because the model will become the cost yardstick for the project. As mentioned earlier, the projected cost analysis of the ambulatory facility should be as comprehensive as possible, reflecting a completed building right down to the sidewalks and utilities to feed it. It should include supporting structures and wiring for radiology equipment, a security system, equipment to wash dishes if a food service area is included, furniture, artwork, and any consultants needed on the project. In short, the cost model is a complete cost picture of the project.
5. A cash flow schedule, which indicates how much money is required and when it is needed throughout the course of the project.
6. A design and construction schedule that details the big steps and the decision points so that everyone can stay on track. This schedule becomes the time yardstick.
7. A code and zoning analysis. This analysis can be brief and should be included to show that the building code and zoning regulations have been reviewed and that they will or will not have an impact on the project.
8. The method that will be used to finance the building and other available options.
9. An operating *pro forma*. This *pro forma* should show the cash flow and income requirements for the operation of the facility and is necessary to test the financial feasibility of the project. When physicians are involved as owners or joint venture partners, they want to know how the venture is going to affect their income over the short term as well as over the long term. Financial feasibility should be looked at unemotionally, taking into account business projections and the additional patient encounters that will be necessary to make the numbers work. A proper statement of space and cost for each department is necessary, as is an assessment of where the patients will come from.
10. A clear statement of what the next steps are going to be should the feasibility study be approved. What happens next, who has responsibility, when will it be done, and how much will it cost?
11. A statement of what decisions are being requested from the board or physicians when they accept this feasibility study.

Critical Points in Design and Construction

In conclusion, the most critical points in the design and construction of the facility include the following:

- To avoid having a much larger building than anticipated, make sure that the space generated in the design phase is always related back to the approved program. Demand that any deviations from this program be accounted for and approved in writing. A little space here and a little space there soon add up to a 5 percent to 10 percent cost overrun.
- Set the cost model, which is based on the services provided, as early as possible, and make sure that the design team accounts for deviations from the model. Always relate the cost model back to the business plan.
- Make sure that the design team provides a schedule for the project and then maintains that schedule throughout the decision-making process.
- Avoid an inpatient atmosphere. Keep the outpatient's comfort and needs at the forefront.
- Insist on materials that will stand up to hard use. The door in a clinic may open 200,000 times in a year.
- Beware of compound fees. If dealing with an architect and several consulting firms, be sure not to pay two or three times for the same service. Always look at the project in terms of the bottom line and relate this back to the business plan.
- Avoid trendy design. Good design is practical and timeless. The building must have an attractive appearance because it is also a marketing tool, but good design and successful business ventures are not mutually exclusive. Next to efficient function, an inviting appearance is most important.
- Understand how the cost per square foot is being calculated and what it includes. Always relate all costs per square foot back to total project cost and to the cost model.
- Have a master plan if the outpatient building is to be integrated into the hospital's campus. If such integration is not done properly, the building can become just another piece of a series of confused parts that confuse the patient and present a distorted image.
- Be decisive. The health care market is competitive and does not wait while someone stalls the decision-making process.

References

1. Lifton, J., and Hardy, O. B. *Site Selection for Health Care Facilities.* Chicago: American Hospital Publishing, Inc., 1982.
2. Lifton and Hardy.

Chapter 5

Integrating Ambulatory Care Expansion with Physicians' Offices

Drexel Toland and Susan Strong

Despite its current growth and public emphasis, ambulatory care has been in existence for as long as patients have been utilizing physicians' offices for treatment. What has changed is that physicians are now competing with hospitals to provide sophisticated facilities in which to perform ambulatory care procedures, and hospitals are competing with physicians for the ambulatory care dollar. As territorial lines and roles blur for hospitals and physicians, new working relationships must be forged that will utilize the talents of both parties as well as meet the public need.

Nowhere can this new relationship develop more logically and effectively than in the natural marriage of the physicians' office building and the ambulatory care center. After all, the physician's office is the original ambulatory care center in any community. Whether located over the drugstore at the turn of the century or in today's modern medical office building on the hospital campus, the physician's office was and still is the primary source of ambulatory care in America. The addition of sophisticated facilities needed to carry out more involved ambulatory care procedures is only a natural outgrowth of that historical function.

Once physicians' offices and ambulatory care centers are combined into an integrated ambulatory care center, the result is a one-stop shopping center for outpatient services. In many instances, the integrated ambulatory care center is located on the hospital campus to act as the central referral hub for outlying primary care and ambulatory services. It houses the hospital's core group of specialists — those physicians who are an integrated and loyal part of the hospital's marketing plan and support system. It is the center of ambulatory care activity, just as the hospital is the center of inpatient treatment.

Whereas the on-campus physicians' office and ambulatory care center is the hub of the hospital's referral system, the spokes radiating from this hub are the outlying primary care physicians and specialists located in private practices, in similar but smaller physicians' office and ambulatory care centers nearby, or in surrounding communities. Some, but not necessarily all, of these physicians will also be a part of the hospital's core group of physicians.

In some cases, a relatively large integrated ambulatory care center is located away from the hospital. This center acts as a major outreach facility to new markets and functions as a feeder of patients into the hospital.

The first step in creating a strong integrated system of ambulatory care is the development of the on-campus ambulatory care center, which is the cornerstone of all other ambulatory care services. The strategic planning that goes into its development will, in turn, direct the hospital to the concomitant development of vital support and referral systems away from the hospital campus.

Planning for Success

The question, then, is how to plan for the successful forging of the physicians' office building and the ambulatory care center into one integrated center for ambulatory care. The planning process can be broken into two basic parts—program and design. Both are essential if the end result is to live up to its full potential. To succeed, executive management must establish program and design goals, research carefully, and program realistically. This approach will likely ensure positive relationships with the medical staff, business success, and financial gain. Adequately designed facilities will mean efficiency and flexibility; satisfied physicians, employees, and patients; and controlled long-range maintenance costs. Overall, success requires diligent planning.

Elements of Successful Planning

The three elements of successful planning are: an understanding of the nature of the project, a method for developing physician support, and an action-oriented, entrepreneurial attitude.

Understanding the Nature of the Project

The first step in successful planning is to arrive at an understanding of the specific nature of the project. For years the debate has raged as to whether an on-campus medical office building should be developed and treated primarily as a real estate venture, or whether it should be treated as an extension of the hospital, not unlike other support departments such as food service, the emergency department, and obstetrics.

The problem with the concept of the real estate venture is that it emphasizes a full building over a building full of the right specialists. Such an emphasis would result in sizing the building according to current demand, rather than according to projected hospital, physician, and community need. It would mean designing the building to turn the best profit, rather than designing it to include special, costly elements, such as soundproofing and individual climate controls in each room, to enhance patients' and physicians' satisfaction over the long term. In short, the concept of the real estate venture addresses the buildings as bricks and mortar, rather than as an implementation tool of the strategic and marketing planning process.

Despite its deceptive similarities to a real estate project, the medical office building can live up to its full potential only when it becomes a part of the integrated planning and development of the hospital as a whole. This concept does not eliminate franchising ownership or operation to others, similar to hiring an outside firm to manage and perform the housekeeping function for the hospital. It does mean maintaining control over the project, its development and operation, and its role in the overall financial and service plan of the hospital. It does not mean eliminating real estate principles entirely, but instead using them as ancillaries to the more important strategic planning to meet hospital, community, and physician needs.

Once integration of ambulatory care services and facilities with the physicians' offices begins, visualization of the whole process as part of strategic planning usually becomes easier. Planning for patient services and facilities traditionally has been a part of a hospital's long-range planning. Vital to the whole process, however, is bringing the physicians' offices into the same context and seeing the whole planning process as one unit—a truly integrated physicians' office and ambulatory care center. This understanding of the basic nature of the process and project is vital to success.

Developing Physician Support

For a project to succeed, it must not only be integrated into the hospital program, but it must also win physicians' support by involving them in ways that help ensure that their needs for income and practice security will be met.

An essential element of success is understanding that without physicians there is neither a need for a hospital and its services nor a mechanism for providing them. The physician is the hospital's distributor. He or she orders the purchase of services for patients. When the hospital works with physicians to help their practices grow and prosper, it is indirectly helping itself to prosper.

Because physicians and hospital management sometimes lack good, cooperative relationships and, in some cases, even have adversarial relationships, it is vital that hospital management understands the importance of the physicians; furthermore, that understanding must precipitate action. The causes of weak relationships, when they exist, must be identified and appropriate action must be taken to solve problems, improve attitudes, and strengthen cooperation.

To work well with their physicians, hospital executives must be intelligent, knowledgeable, and enthusiastic. They must do their homework and know what they are talking about. They must be willing to take a stand on issues and act decisively. Management must also show respect for its medical staff members and deal with them honestly and forthrightly. Management must be willing to listen to the physicians. Failure in any of these areas can greatly hamper relationships with physicians and support for the project.

The physicians must be included in project planning from the very beginning. Determining the specific needs and problems of the medical staff and finding ways to meet those needs and solve those problems are essential parts of planning. Without the physicians' ideas and opinions, physician support is very difficult to obtain.

For best results, the inclusion of physicians in the planning process should be structured. Physicians should be given an opportunity to express their views in one-on-one, confidential interviews. In addition, an advisory committee representing the medical staff in matters that affect the staff should be an official part of the planning team.[1]

No ambulatory care program will succeed without the support of the medical staff, and evidence of hospital management's desire to help the physicians will help to gain that support. In short, to secure medical staff support, hospital executives must approach the physicians with attitudes of respect, demonstrate support for their needs as relationships are developed, and include the physicians in project planning.

Having an Action-Oriented, Entrepreneurial Attitude

To succeed in today's market, hospital executives must be action-oriented and have an entrepreneurial attitude. Although hospital executives often work under far more constraints than the typical entrepreneur, they must, nonetheless, adopt at least some of the entrepreneurial spirit: they must be willing to make tough, timely decisions; to take risks, and to act.

Of course, adequate study must precede appropriate decision making and action. However, time and time again projects have been studied, discussed, planned, and postponed for three, five, or even more years. The result is that the hospital misses opportunities and loses credibility with the medical staff. The cause of the delay is usually management's fear of the medical staff's dissension or opposition.

The best cure for that situation is for hospital management to determine the hospital's needs, establish goals, prepare a plan of action, and then meet with the medical staff to get their opinions, ideas, and assistance. It is management's responsibility to determine what the hospital will undertake.

It is the physicians' contribution to help determine the best way to do it—for the physicians and their patients.

Consideration of the physicians' needs and desires in the planning process is essential to success. However, the hospital executive must never lose sight of the fact that physicians are in the business of practicing medicine, not running hospitals. Just as the hospital can help its physicians enhance their practices, physicians can help hospital management plan more effectively. Hospital management, however, is ultimately responsible for making decisions concerning the hospital's future and for acting on them.

Program Planning

Good, productive, careful program planning to ensure the success of the project is made up of a number of elements: determination of hospital needs and goals, formulation of the medical staff profile and master plan, market research, consideration of all the options, business plan development, and program development. In short, administrators must determine the needs of the hospital, the medical staff, and the community; consider all the options for meeting those needs; determine what is feasible to carry out; and identify the tasks and time frames needed to complete the project. The process is that simple. What is not simple is the many detailed steps in accomplishing this planning.

Hospital Needs and Goals

Focusing clearly on hospital needs and goals is essential for determining the best way to meet them. As obvious as that statement is, it is still frequently ignored. For example, mixed motives often blur planning vision. A clear vision of what the hospital wants to accomplish through the development of an integrated ambulatory care center is essential to success. It includes strategic planning and specific goal setting. In the process, many questions must be answered. Is the hospital's goal to increase inpatient admissions? Does the hospital want to replace inpatient income with ambulatory care income? Is the ambulatory care project being considered primarily as a means of developing physician loyalty? Is its goal market penetration into a rapidly growing area? What other motives does the hospital management have?

The answers to these questions profoundly affect the integrated ambulatory care center. On the one hand, if the hospital's goal is to increase inpatient admissions, not all ambulatory care services in the center necessarily need to produce profit. The center may generate numerous inpatient referrals, and hence will still be of great financial benefit to the hospital even though it may be only a break-even (or less) operation on its own. On the other hand, if the generation of income on the ambulatory care level to replace lost inpatient income is more important to the hospital, each service considered for the ambulatory care center needs to be examined carefully for the number of dollars it can generate. In turn, the specialists selected to occupy the physicians' offices will need to complement specifically the ambulatory care services and programs offered, and outlying support systems should be planned accordingly.

In addition to these questions, others also must be addressed during the goal-setting process. What are the hospital's financial parameters; for example, limits and goals? What can the hospital afford to do? What will it have difficulty capitalizing? What information does management need to share with physicians in order to obtain their support? These answers may not only affect the size and scope of the project, but also may determine, at least partially, how specific aspects of the project are organized.

Medical Staff Profile and Master Plan

Once goals and parameters have been established, management should begin researching the medical staff profile and master plan. This area of planning is one of the most essential to the future of the integrated physicians' office and ambulatory care center, as well as to the future viability of the hospital. The results of the medical staff research will significantly influence the course of the project and may even cause changes in the hospital's goals.

The major objectives of the medical staff profile and master plan include the following:

1. To inventory the physician supply both on the hospital staff and in the primary service area
2. To analyze the medical staff to determine its current and projected support for the hospital
3. To determine the number and types of physicians needed on the hospital staff and in the primary service area
4. To create a master plan that projects the number and specialties of physicians needed on the hospital staff in the future with regard to current and projected services, current and projected support from the physicians, and service area need

In short, the medical staff profile and master plan examines supply and demand and projects niches to be filled and needs to be met. It is the road map for developing sufficient physician support for successful ambulatory care programs as well as inpatient admissions. Typical elements of the medical staff profile and master plan that should be examined include the following:

1. *Inventory of medical staff membership.* The inventory of medical staff membership includes a head count of physicians by subspecialty in each staff category—active, associate, courtesy, honorary, and such—in order to get a clear picture of current medical staff membership.
2. *Medical staff specialty distribution over a five-year period.* By looking at medical staff membership by specialty over a five-year period, hospital management can determine areas of strong or weak growth and spot indications of problems. For example, failure to have a substantial number of associate or probationary physicians move up to active staff status may indicate deficiencies in programs, facilities, or relationships or that competing hospitals are doing a better job of securing associate or probationary physicians' loyalty.
3. *Admissions by specialty over a five-year period, including percentages.* These figures indicate broad trends—areas of growing and dropping admissions and changes in the percentage of total admissions contributed by each specialty. Some changes will reflect trends toward ambulatory care; others will indicate potentially growing or dropping market share; and still others will signal potential problems to be investigated further.
4. *Admissions by subspecialty over a five-year period, including patterns of each physician admitting.* Examination of the admitting patterns of each physician and, collectively, each group of subspecialists reveals considerable constructive data. It clearly indicates strong and weak areas of admissions. It reveals dropping admitting patterns to be evaluated further on the basis of impact of ages of the physicians, the shifts to outpatient care, and possible problems with or shifts in loyalty. It pinpoints areas of growth and potential growth that also should be analyzed on the basis of age, likely outpatient shifts, and the potential for continued support and loyalty. Invariably this examination will produce some surprising results as well as confirm previously suspected strengths and weaknesses.
5. *Average number of admissions per physician by specialty over a five-year period.* As average admissions per physician drop on a national scale, examination of average admissions of the hospital's staff shows how well the medical staff or hospital is faring by comparison. Parallel drops may only indicate that average admissions are in line with the rest of the country. Accelerated drops might indicate, among other things, that physicians are shifting their admissions to other hospitals. Strongly increasing admissions might indicate growth of market share or reflect the results of appropriate recruiting or practice enhancement programs.
6. *Profile of the top 20 admitting physicians.* A look at the top 20 admitting physicians, their subspecialties, total admissions, and ages can

be quite revealing. Usually, these 20 physicians produce a particularly high percentage of total admissions. Their ages may indicate whether to expect further increases or declines in admissions. Their specialties are probably ones that usually generate higher-than-average admissions, such as internal medicine and cardiology. However, even this analysis may reveal surprises that can cue the hospital to market potential. The total admissions of these 20 physicians can indicate how vulnerable the hospital is with regard to their continued support.

7. *Average age of physicians by subspecialty.* Because American Medical Association (AMA) statistics show that physician productivity normally increases into middle age and then begins to decline until retirement, age is a very important indicator in projecting future support from a hospital's medical staff. A look at the average age of each subspecialty group tells hospital management which subspecialties are particularly vulnerable to future declines in admissions and outright retirements. It also indicates which areas have strong potential for the future.

8. *Age distribution of the medical staff as compared to national averages.* Further indication of the significance of the staff's age distribution comes from comparing it with national averages. On the one hand, a medical staff that has more physicians in the older age categories than the national average often needs an aggressive recruitment program. On the other hand, a hospital with a very young staff may want to emphasize practice enhancement and building relationships with and benefits for its staff members.

9. *Age distribution and admissions activity of the medical staff.* An analysis of age distribution and admissions activity of the medical staff divides the staff into five-year age increments — 40 and under, 41–45, 46–50, and so forth. Each increment is then examined according to the number of physicians within the group, each group's admissions, the percentage of the physicians on the staff in each group, and their percentage of total admissions. Such an analysis shows which age group is contributing the largest absolute number of admissions as well as which age groups are contributing more or less than their relative shares of admissions. Managers can determine whether admissions are growing appropriately with age into the peak admitting years and then declining, or if potential problems are being revealed by abnormal trends.

10. *Average admissions by physician age.* An analysis of average admissions by physician age gives further confirmation of the data previously described. Again, such analysis should show an admissions curve appropriate for the age categories. If it does not, further research is needed to determine why.

11. *Age distribution of physicians admitting above-average numbers of patients.* A final look at age indicates in which categories the above-average admitters are located. Again, it should confirm previous data as well as show the percentage of total admissions these physicians produce. Quite often, a very few physicians produce the majority of hospital admissions.

12. *Population-to-physician ratios for the United States as a whole and for metropolitan areas, states, and the primary service area (PSA) of the hospital, as well as the optimum ratio for the PSA.* Whereas previous data have profiled the medical staff, the physician-to-population ratios put the hospital and its staff into perspective within the primary service area. This element of the medical staff profile shows the ratio of population per physician by subspecialty for the nation as a whole, for metropolitan areas, for the state in which the hospital is located, for the primary service area, and for optimum business in the PSA. These ratios are developed by using the best available government and AMA data.

13. *Physician manpower needs by subspecialty for the primary service area.* A comparison of the number of physicians already practicing within the PSA with the various ratios indicated in the population-to-physician data indicates the number or range of physicians needed in the PSA. These numbers represent indicators, not absolutes. The demographics of the PSA must come into play as ranges are narrowed to more specific numbers.

14. *Projections of medical staff manpower needed to achieve optimum utilization of the hospital.* In order to create a master plan of physicians to be considered the core group of specialists for the hospital, hospital programs and needs must be considered. An analysis of the current average number of admissions per physician, the number of operating beds, the average length of stay, and the desired occupancy level determines the general number of physicians needed to achieve that occupancy. This analysis can be further refined by breaking that total number down by hospital service. For the purposes of ambulatory care, the analysis would need to be evaluated on the basis of outpatient procedure statistics. Finally, for the projections to be valid, adjustments must be made to anticipate future trends or events for the time period for which projections are made. For example, if average inpatient admissions are dropping and outpatient procedures are rising, those trends must be factored in. Similarly, the projected addition or deletion of beds or services must also be considered. The end result is a physician manpower goal for the hospital—the total number of physicians needed to support hospital beds and services at the desired level of utilization.

15. *Projected physician manpower needs by subspecialty for the hospital
    for a five-year period.* Finally, outlining a medical staff master plan
    for the hospital requires a refinement of the physician manpower
    goal into projections for a five-year period of the number of phy-
    sicians in each subspecialty needed to support the hospital. The
    first step in making these projections is to set physician manpower
    goals by subspecialty. These goals take into consideration the opti-
    mum number of physicians in each subspecialty, tempered by any
    idiosyncrasies of the PSA and programs emphasized by the hospi-
    tal. These numbers are then adjusted by the current number of phy-
    sicians on the staff and the number of physicians aged 60 or over
    who will be cutting back their practices and possibly retiring over
    the next five years. The physician manpower goals indicate the mix-
    ture of specialties the hospital would like to have on staff. The
    adjusted numbers tell the hospital which specialists it needs to attract
    in order to meet those goals. The manpower needs of the PSA indi-
    cate whether specialists need to be recruited from outside the PSA
    or whether they are already available but practicing at nearby
    hospitals.

In addition to the analyses described above, further analysis is needed
to totally integrate ambulatory care into the medical staff master-planning
process. Many hospitals have not kept adequate records to determine the
number of outpatient procedures or admissions generated by each physician. As patient services continue to shift into the ambulatory care arena,
however, such data are becoming increasingly more important and should
now be a standard part of hospital record keeping.

When outpatient data are available, the medical staff master plan should
include them in its analysis. Items numbered 3, 4, 5, 6, 9, 10, and 11 in the
preceding pages should include both inpatient admissions analysis and outpatient procedures analysis. These data are particularly important for the
hospital trying to determine which ambulatory care services have the greatest
potential and should be considered for incorporation into the integrated
physicians' office and ambulatory care center.

In addition, because inpatient admissions and outpatient procedures
can vary so widely in their financial contribution to the hospital, an additional analysis of gross or net income generated per physician for the hospital
can also be a valuable tool. However, caution must be exercised to ensure
that financial numbers do not become the primary parameters of medical
staff planning.

A balanced mixture of specialists is essential to keeping a medical staff
working smoothly. Many hospitals today already have physicians located
on the hospital campus, but other hospitals have medical staffs that are formally organized in a large group practice or clinics that operate separately

from the independent physicians. In either case, a market share analysis of on-campus versus off-campus physicians or clinic physicians versus independent physicians can also be valuable in establishing a medical staff master plan. These additional analyses can shed further light on hospital and medical staff strengths and weaknesses that must be considered in planning.

Market Research

Market research looks at the community to determine which services, programs, and facilities are provided where. It searches for unmet or inadequately met needs. It also studies the community's desire for services, as well as what physicians believe is needed and how they want those needs to be met. From this research comes a picture of niches to be filled and potential market needs to be met.

Examination of population-to-physician ratios and other elements of the medical staff master plan were the first steps in developing market research. Other steps must follow.

With regard to the physicians' offices, market research should include an inventory of other physicians' office buildings in town, occupancy levels, rental rates and services included in the rents, number of condominiums or other physician-owned buildings, and level of satisfaction of physicians located in these facilities. This information will help facility planners develop a building that is appropriate to the market in which it is located. It will also identify characteristics needed to give a competitive edge to the facility being planned. A word of caution: because of the unique nature of on-campus offices, absorption rates should not be overemphasized in planning the building.

In order to determine ambulatory care services needed and desired in the primary service area, the hospital planning staff or its consultants should begin by looking at demographic characteristics. This research may already have been completed as a part of the hospital's long-range strategic plan or marketing plan, but the data need careful examination in relation to ambulatory services planning. Typical demographic characteristics that give clues to the services needed are age, sex, family size, race or ethnic origin, income, housing, education, occupation, unemployment and employment rates, and vehicles per household. The following list explains why these characteristics are important:

1. *Age.* Age characteristics of a population being served can offer many suggestions as to appropriate services. For example, according to the AMA, elderly patients use more services provided by primary care physicians, radiologists, and surgeons than other people do. In addition, adults have more surgery than children. Thus, a community with a very young population may need fewer surgical services than

a service area with more elderly people. Programs such as day-care centers for those with Alzheimer's disease and other age-related services may also be successful among the elderly. However, an elderly population may be resistant to change, which must be considered when moving services from inpatient to outpatient settings. A young population may indicate a need for fast services and treatment facilities.

2. *Sex.* The sex characteristics of a population add still further information about the types of outpatient services to be considered. Even when childbearing is taken out of consideration, women still use more health care services than men. If a large segment of the population is composed of females in their childbearing years, additional utilization of services is indicated. Many women's services and women's centers have been developed in response to this important market. In addition, females make more of the health care decisions than males, even for others. Thus, services that appeal to females and meet their needs are particularly significant.

3. *Family size.* A population with large families usually is very concerned with the cost of health care. Consequently, areas with large families may actually experience lower utilization per capita than similar populations of small family units. Emphasis on basics delivered economically may be an appropriate thrust in areas of large family size.

4. *Race or ethnic origin.* According to the AMA, certain racial or ethnic groups see physicians less frequently and rely instead on clinics and hospital emergency departments. Because these individuals are less likely to get preventive care, their need for services when they do seek medical care is often more acute. With such ethnic groups, economic conditions often play a part in which services they use. In addition, language can be a barrier with some ethnic groups. Taking into consideration these special needs could greatly influence the types of ambulatory services provided by a hospital with large ethnic constituencies.

5. *Income.* High-income populations can afford a variety of services that low-income populations cannot. The higher the income, however, the less often the individual tends to see the physician for a scheduled visit. According to the AMA, high-income individuals use hospital emergency departments and outpatient services less often than others. One might conclude that lower-income individuals put off care, are sicker when they seek it, and need low-cost alternatives, whereas higher-income individuals are more oriented toward prevention and utilize services with more amenities when they do seek care.

6. *Housing.* Housing can provide still other clues as to the types of services that are needed and will be used. On one end of the spectrum,

if the population is transient — an average of less than five years in current housing — it is more likely to use walk-in clinics and to have no regular physicians. On the other end of the spectrum, if housing is rather old and little new construction is going on in the area, the population is probably aging with the housing that exists. The more stable the population, the more likely the residents are to have established relationships with physicians.

7. *Education.* A high educational level is an excellent indicator for possible utilization of ambulatory care services. With higher education comes the use of more specialists, more emphasis on preventive care, and greater expenditures on health care. In short, a high level of education is an indicator of a strong target market. These are the people to whom wellness programs, radiology screening programs, and other similar services will appeal most.

8. *Occupation.* Occupation, education, and income are closely related to one another. Occupation does, however, tend to reflect social class more than any other indicator. On the one hand, if the hospital is serving a largely white-collar work force, education and income are usually high, and ambulatory care services oriented toward preventive care, specialty services, and stress are likely to be successful. On the other hand, if the work force is largely blue-collar, a greater need for occupational medical programs geared toward accidental injury and workplace environmental problems may well be indicated.

9. *Unemployment and employment rates.* High unemployment rates ultimately create health care problems. Unemployed individuals tend to put off treatment and to be in greater need when treatment is sought. Services that would appeal to high-income areas would have a low probability of doing well when unemployment rates are high. However, when rates of employment are high, particularly when a large percentage of households have two employed heads of household, certain needs will be dictated — especially the need for flexible hours and services. Child care for sick children is in greater demand when both parents are working, and these households will also put a high premium on convenience, such as having OB/GYN services and pediatric services in one location. Two-income households will also have more money to spend on health care that meets their special needs.

10. *Vehicles per household.* The number of vehicles per household not only reflects income and life-style, but may also indicate the need for accessibility to public transportation in areas where the number of vehicles is low.

This list is not all-inclusive, and other demographic characteristics may be added. For example, in areas where military bases are located, the demographic data should take into account that many of the military personnel and their families will be using health care services provided by the military rather than the community.

Besides demographic data, health care utilization data are of critical importance. Although most service areas will fall into normal ranges of incidence of disease and injuries, other areas are at high risk. For example, orthopedic injuries are high in Hawaii, where many surfing accidents take place; and lung diseases will usually be more prevalent in mining areas. Familiarity with health care utilization statistics of an area can provide added insight into potential ambulatory care services.

In addition, careful examination of hospital inpatient and outpatient utilization data by service and procedure reveals areas in which the hospital is already building a market and uncovers areas of further potential. Services that are suitable for outpatient delivery, that can be provided as efficiently or more efficiently on an outpatient basis, and that can be provided more economically on an ambulatory basis should certainly be considered for the integrated ambulatory care center. However, moving a service from inpatient to outpatient status can sometimes mean a lower profit per case for the hospital. But if the service is provided more attractively and more economically for the patient on an outpatient basis, the change should be considered despite lower profit. Eventually, competition will dictate the switch, and the hospital that takes a leadership position has the opportunity to capture a greater market share.

Although demographic and health care utilization data both provide the statistical information needed to determine which ambulatory care services should be considered, two other bodies of data must be considered before the market research is completed. These are consumer preference data and physician preference data.

Despite all the possible niches that statistical data can reveal, if consumers are not interested in an ambulatory service or are not willing to pay for a service, particularly if it is elective, they will not use it, and so the development of such a service can be disastrous. As planning progresses, surveying a sample of the market for general areas of need and dissatisfaction as well as for specific service details can be extremely important.

An equally important element of a successful ambulatory care service is physician interest in either providing or referring to the service. Careful discussions with medical staff members to determine their interest can provide valuable information on which services to pursue first and which services are likely to be successful.

Obviously, not all staff members need to be interested in a particular service for it to be included in the integrated physicians' office and ambulatory care center, but the appropriate number and types of specialists must be interested. For example, a commercial service such as optical dispensing would only be appropriate in a center that had ophthalmologists who were interested in referring to it. Although a weight-loss clinic might be successful just by marketing directly to the consumer market, it can be even more successful if it has strong referral support from physicians. An ambulatory surgery service would not be successful if all the surgeons already owned such a service and refused to use the one in the center.

Market research is a relatively new field for hospitals. It is vital, however, to the successful development of an integrated ambulatory care center. By combining careful examination of demographic data, health care utilization data, consumer preference data, and physician interest data, the hospital or its consultants can begin formulating a list of potential ambulatory care and commercial services to be included in the integrated ambulatory care center.

Service Offerings

The list of ambulatory services that can be included in an integrated ambulatory care center is very long. New services are initiated daily by creative and competitive hospitals. Whereas services could once be divided conveniently into such categories as hospital-provided, ambulatory care, and commercial services, today commercial providers have moved into areas that were once considered the hospital's domain, and the lines of distinction are no longer clear.

In an integrated ambulatory care center, services are likely to fall into three categories—those that are an extension of physicians' practices, those that are an extension of hospital services, and those that are strictly commercial. Many of the services could fall into any of these categories, depending on the individual situation. For example, whereas a laboratory may once have been run by the hospital, it may now be operated by a commercial laboratory. A cardiac rehabilitation program may be part of a physician's practice, may be an extension of the cardiac rehabilitation services of the hospital, or may be owned by licensed technicians who operate it independently. Only such services as a satellite bank teller might clearly be considered commercial today.

Among the many ambulatory care services that could be considered for an integrated ambulatory care center are the following:

- Laboratory
- Imaging center, including many combinations of services
- Ambulatory surgery, laser surgery
- Women's center
- Wellness programs, including fitness, sports medicine, and prenatal fitness
- Weight-control clinic for chronic obesity or cosmetic purposes
- Cancer treatment center

- Rehabilitation — cardiac or physical
- Geriatric services, health education, and adult day care
- Pediatric services, including sick-child day care and enuresis (bed-wetting) treatment
- Occupational health clinic/urgent care clinic
- Diabetes treatment center
- Pain center
- Drug and alcohol dependency program
- Psychological counseling and group therapy programs, such as stress management and relaxation training, and programs for depression, premenstrual syndrome, divorce recovery, and teen pregnancy
- Hemodialysis
- Dermatology clinic and psoriasis treatment center
- Sexual impotence treatment
- Smoking cessation program
- Other services of a more commercial nature, such as the following:
  - Pharmacy
  - Hotel facilities
  - Gift shop
  - Flower shop
  - Durable medical goods
  - Home health services
  - Optical dispensary
  - Branch bank
  - Coffee shop/restaurant/vending snack shop
  - Uniform shop
  - Photograph developing
  - Laundry/dry cleaner
  - Bakery

Not all commercial businesses located within an integrated ambulatory care center will be highly profitable, any more than one can say that all fast-food franchises will be successful when they open in a city. In the fast-food industry, McDonald's has an awesome track record because the company has strict service and marketing standards. It does its homework before opening a new franchise.

The same kind of research used for such commercial enterprises as McDonald's can help determine the need for services to be located in an integrated ambulatory care center. No simple formula exists for saying which will do well and which will not. Each situation is unique, and careful market research will direct the hospital to the services it should include.

As the hospital considers which services it will include in the integrated ambulatory care center, it should avoid the common error of limiting its consideration to services that only the hospital or its medical staff is capable of providing. An integrated ambulatory care center can function very effectively with franchised operations in it. "Reinventing the wheel" is foolish if the hospital can enlist established firms with track records to provide some of the special services. Frequently, a national or regional firm can contribute much greater expertise and economy of scale than the hospital can to the development and operation of a service and, consequently, may be much more price competitive. By working with proprietary firms, the hospital may be able to provide a much more complete array of services than would otherwise be possible.

A variety of ownership or joint venture packages can be developed among hospitals, physicians, and independent providers to enable the hospital or physicians or both to share in the earnings from the opportunities provided in the integrated physicians' office and ambulatory care centers. The wise hospital will consider all the options carefully before proceeding.

After examining all the available options and applying the market research to those options, the hospital will be able to develop a narrowed list of services to be considered for the physicians' office and ambulatory care center. The next step is to examine further each of those options to determine their specific viability.

Business Plans

For each ambulatory care service being considered for the joint facility, a separate business plan should be developed. It should include detailed market research information to confirm the demand for the service and its projected usage. Much of this research will have already taken place, but at this point product- or service-specific consumer and physician research is required. What is the competition for this service (if any)? Who is providing it, where, and at what price? Who will use this service? What are they willing to pay for it? What features will make the service more attractive, especially more attractive than competing services (if any)? How often will the service be used? Will physicians be providing the service? If so, are they interested? What will it take to secure their cooperation? Will the service need referrals from physicians? If so, will they refer to it? What will be needed in services, structure, and incentives to secure physician cooperation? These types of specifics must be addressed in order to determine the real need for the service and how it should be provided.

Once the demand is established, the business plan should outline the size and type of space needed to meet that projected demand. The plan should also include a detailed ownership and operational structure, information about how the service will be financed, and a pro forma statement for at least the first year and preferably for the first three to five years of operation. If a joint venture is involved, it should spell out who will be involved and how the venture will be structured, how earnings and losses will be distributed, and how the venture can be dissolved or how a member can exit from it.

There are many companies that do business planning. Unless a hospital has strong experience in this area, it may want to hire one of these companies in order to develop not only a thorough plan but also an objective one. Only after a business plan is completed for a specific service will the hospital be able to determine its feasibility and whether it is to be included in the integrated ambulatory care center.

Program Development

From the medical staff master plan comes the first step in developing the program for the integrated physicians' office and ambulatory care center. This step includes determining the number and types of specialists to be included in the building.

Obviously, not all medical staff members will be located on campus. Usually, the hospital building will have a stronger emphasis on specialists and subspecialists than on primary care physicians, but that is not always appropriate. The marketing plan of the hospital should be taken into consideration as the decision is made with regard to the specialties to be located on campus and those to be located in outlying areas.

Undoubtedly, the marketing plan will have looked at physicians' office locations as well as patient origins for the whole community. The plan will have uncovered prime target areas to capture growing markets or to fill unmet needs. Many of the primary care physicians will be located in these outlying locations, as well as obstetricians, gynecologists, pediatricians, internists, orthopedists, and ophthalmologists.

Strong referral ties with these outlying physicians are vital, but first the hospital must establish its on-campus hub. The on-campus facility should include a balanced mixture of physicians, based on the overall manpower goals of the hospital. The facility should include room for current medical staff members who want to be located in the building, as well as room for physicians who will need to be added to the staff. Ultimately, the hospital usually will want 50 to 75 percent of its core group of physicians to be located on the hospital campus.

The almost universal tendency is for planners to underestimate the demand for space in this building that will arise once it is under way. Consequently, programming sufficient space is vital. Usually only about one-third of the physicians who will ultimately occupy the center will express interest in locating there during the planning stages. (For more details on programming physician occupancy, see *Hospital-Based Medical Office Buildings.*[2])

Once the hospital has determined the total number of physicians who will have offices in the integrated ambulatory care center, it should estimate approximately 1,000 square feet of space per physician in the building to determine the space requirements for physician tenants.

After completing market research and business plans for each of the ambulatory care and commercial services being considered for the building, the hospital will then need to decide which services to program for the building. Because the individual business plans for the services will include space needs based on projected demand, these needs can simply be totaled for a program of services and space in the ambulatory care sector.

In addition, the hospital may want to consider any other inclusions for the integrated ambulatory care center, such as hospital offices or teaching facilities that it might want to relocate from the hospital. Once these facilities (if any) have been added to the list, the program of tenants and space is complete, and the project can move to the design phase.

Architectural Planning and Design

Functional and effective design is essential to a successful project. Many of the elements that enter into an appropriate design are discussed in chapter 4. However, several key elements are worthy of special emphasis.

Hospital planners must realize that as health care moves from the inpatient arena to the ambulatory arenas, patients have more choices. Patients choose their physicians and frequently participate in the selection of their own treatment. For this reason, function alone will not meet the architectural needs of the physicians' office and ambulatory care center.

To attract patients to the physicians and to walk-in types of services, the center must be more than a building that merely does the job; it also must invite the patient's presence. The strictly functional design of hospitals from years past must be forgotten. Instead, hospitals must begin to think in terms of comfort and visual amenities. The integrated ambulatory care center should be the most attractive building on the hospital campus.

Campus Zoning

An important step in establishing the building's unique and attractive appearance while integrating its multiple functions is zoning the hospital campus. No longer can the hospital campus afford to be a maze of confusing buildings if it is to function effectively and attract patients to the ambulatory care facilities. The campus should be zoned into four areas: in-hospital acute facilities; ambulatory care facilities; other facilities, such as extended- or life-care areas; and parking. The key to effective design is making these areas work with and be convenient to one another. By zoning the campus, an attractive, inviting integrated ambulatory care center can be developed.

Ten characteristics should be considered for locating the ambulatory care zone:

1. *Distinct identity.* Ambulatory care facilities should be easily recognizable as an entity separate from the inpatient facilities. Having ambulatory care services in a separate building provides not only a stronger identity, but also a friendlier atmosphere that attracts patients. This reduces the fear often associated with the hospital itself. In addition, the location of the ambulatory services should be highly visible in order to make it easy for patients to find them and to remind patients of their availability.

2. *Physical connection to the hospital.* Physicians' offices and ambulatory care facilities should be close enough to be physically connected to the hospital by an enclosed walkway, bridge, or tunnel. This is especially important because the ambulatory care facilities may include imaging or testing equipment that may be used by inpatients. Failure to connect the two facilities limits their flexibility.

3. *Easy accessibility.* The ambulatory care zone should be located so that a walkway can directly link the diagnostic testing areas of the hospital with the ambulatory care facilities of the center. Easy movement both of patients and physicians from one facility to another is very important. In addition, for greatest utilization of commercial services, pedestrian traffic flow should be routed past them on the way to the hospital.

4. *Convenient parking.* The ambulatory care zone must be convenient to the parking zone. Convenience is very important to ambulatory care patients.

5. *Smooth traffic flow.* Both vehicular and pedestrian traffic must be able to flow in and out of the ambulatory care zone smoothly. It is preferable for each kind of traffic to have a separate entrance to the ambulatory care facility.

6. *Compatibility with the hospital.* The ambulatory care facilities must not interfere with future expansion or redesign of the hospital.

7. *Provision for expansion.* The ambulatory care zone should be sufficiently large to allow for future expansion of its facilities. In addition, those facilities should be located so as to facilitate that expansion, particularly in light of ambulatory care growth.

8. *Land availability.* Sufficient land must either be owned by the hospital or available for purchase. Long-range planning is extremely important in land acquisition and utilization. Failure to plan for future land needs and to utilize available land judiciously can cost the hospital millions of dollars in the long run.

9. *Minimal site improvements.* The site selected for the ambulatory care zone should require a minimum of improvements in order to build on it, for all improvements will add to the cost of construction.

10. *Pleasing aesthetics.* As previously mentioned, the visual appearance of ambulatory facilities and the ambulatory care zone is very important. The site must be aesthetically pleasing, and all construction should encourage the patient to want to be there. It should be the most attractive and least institutional-looking part of the hospital campus.

Design Elements

In addition to campus zoning, specific design elements of the integrated physicians' office and ambulatory care facilities are important to the success of the project. High-quality, functional, attractive facilities can provide a competitive edge in a consumer market that is becoming increasingly quality-conscious. Obviously, without specialists who are recognized for their high-quality practice of medicine, no physicians' office and ambulatory care center can project a high-quality image. However, once the medical staff is developed, the level of quality of the facilities and their maintenance are equated with the level of quality of the medical care in the minds of the patients.

The following four design characteristics are especially important to high-quality construction and physician and patient satisfaction over the long term:

1. *Extra sound control.* Medical buildings require extra sound control so that private conversations taking place in one room cannot be heard in the next. Extra insulation, special treatment of air ducts and handling systems, the staggered placement of electrical outlets, and other similar steps must be taken to ensure this control.
2. *Multiple zoning of heating, ventilating, and air-conditioning (HVAC) systems.* It is essential in integrated ambulatory care centers that systems be zoned so that sick and disrobed patients can be kept comfortably warm and work stations and offices can be kept comfortably cool. Not only must systems be quiet, but they also must provide sufficient exchange of air to remove unpleasant odors. In addition, HVAC systems must be carefully designed so that ducts do not transmit sound from one room to the next, causing loss of privacy.
3. *Efficient elevators.* In a multistory building, nothing causes more consternation than waiting for elevators. Neither busy doctors nor disabled patients want to wait for elevators. Consequently, elevator service must be ample, rapid, and large enough to handle at least an ambulance stretcher, and have a minimum of one elevator capable of handling a hospital gurney.
4. *Convenient and ample parking.* Convenient and ample parking is another essential element of a high-quality facility. Vehicles should

be able to drive under a covered area to let out patients and proceed directly to a nearby parking area. Some areas even offer valet parking for added convenience. Convenient parking for physicians and staff is also important to keep the tenants happy. Six to eight parking spaces should be planned for each physician located in the office building, with parking added for each ambulatory service according to its projected caseload.

Conclusion

The integration of physicians' offices with ambulatory care facilities is a natural combination that results in convenience both for patients and physicians. The process of integrating the facilities involves much research, careful planning, good decisions, and a certain amount of instinct to lead the hospital into an effective and successful project. The benefits in potential income, market strength, and referrals to the hospital can certainly make the effort worthwhile. In fact, the hospital of the future may well be a large integrated physicians' office and ambulatory care center with a small building connected to it to house the high-technology inpatient services.

References

1. Toland, D., and Strong, S. *Hospital-Based Medical Office Buildings.* Chicago: American Hospital Publishing, Inc., 1986.

2. Toland and Strong, pp. 147–48.

Chapter 6

Technological Considerations

Theodore A. Matson

Advances in medical technology can have significant effects on the cost of patient care, reduce lengths of stay, alter the inpatient and outpatient mix, and affect staffing complements of health professionals. Technology has been, and will continue to be, a major driving force in health care delivery. Today, the technology environment offers tremendous opportunities for improved diagnosis and treatment of patients. Although the new technology has been hailed as contributing greatly to advances in medicine, it also has been criticized for its perceived role in increasing health care costs. As hospitals strive to acquire new and improved technologies, those technologies will be scrutinized for their role in enhancing health outcomes.

In the past, major technologies have emerged for inpatient-related activities. With the advent of prospective payment systems and the shifting of care to outpatient settings, the future of technologies will become a major focus of the ambulatory care environment. Hospitals will face a continuous challenge in this area, because new technologies will be widespread and will alter traditional methods of health care delivery. Obtaining capital to acquire these modalities will be increasingly difficult; acquisitions will have to be prioritized according to institutional commitment and marketplace needs. Still, the coming years will be an exciting period of major change in which to participate.

The New Technology Era

Today's delivery of health care services is primarily a result of technological developments during the past 20 years—the new technology era. These developments have dramatically altered the manner in which services are delivered, as well as the practice and staffing patterns of physicians and health personnel. Although it originally focused on equipment concerns, the definition of technology is now broad-based, encompassing not only equipment that provides diagnostic evaluations and therapies, but also new techniques, medical and surgical procedures, pharmaceuticals, and devices.

With this definition in mind, it is conceivable that future technological advancements will shape significant strategies in ambulatory care development over the next decade. The diffusion of medical technology is already becoming widespread. For instance, cardiac catheterizations were once performed exclusively on an inpatient basis. Currently, they represent one of the fastest-growing outpatient procedures in hospitals. It is predicted that over 50 percent of these procedures will soon be performed on an outpatient basis. [1]

In addition to the relocation of former inpatient procedures to the outpatient setting, the new era of technology is bringing about services only envisioned several years ago. For instance, new reproductive technologies, such as in vitro fertilization and gamete intrafallopian transfer, have been developed to treat infertility. Some proponents predict that up to 20 percent of pregnancies in the United States will be conceived through some form of reproductive technology. [2] As another example, newly developed biotherapeutic drugs will be an important development in the fight against cancer. As these drugs are adopted, they increasingly will be provided in the outpatient setting and will no doubt influence the mix and delivery of care to outpatients.

Although new advances will create diversification options in ambulatory care programming, the greatest impact of technological advancement in the short term will be the continuing refinement of existing medical technologies. Providers have become accustomed to enhancements of these technologies; but although manufacturers are willing to pay incremental costs for enhancements, they often are reluctant to invest substantial monies on unproven ideas. Multiple generations of medical technology are evident in the many updated versions of computed tomography (CT) and magnetic resonance imaging (MRI).

Overall, the technology movement will offer a competitive edge in providing new and improved services both for inpatients and outpatients. Despite concerns that technology significantly increases the cost of care, patients today desire high-tech medicine because it represents an important element in their perception of high-quality care. Because of the strong consumer orientation in the health care delivery system and the necessity to provide cutting-edge services, ambulatory care will continue to be driven by technological enhancement and change.

Technologies That Affect Ambulatory Care

The long-term value of technology appears to be its ability to replace expensive inpatient procedures and admissions with care delivered in less-costly ambulatory settings. As technological advances allow more procedures to be performed on an ambulatory basis, the challenge for hospital executives will be to select the most appropriate mix of services consistent with marketplace needs. Priorities for technology must be established because all services cannot be acquired or exploited by a single institution. As strategies are developed for long-term service positioning, it is important to understand the major technologies that will increasingly affect ambulatory care. Although decisions affecting technology will not always focus on ambulatory care considerations, it is clear that the outpatient setting will be the location of choice for technology in the future.

Cardiac Catheterization

Today, cardiology services, including cardiac catheterization, are increasingly being performed on an outpatient basis. Cardiac catheterization is a diagnostic procedure that allows visualization of the coronary arteries in order to detect blockages of blood flow and cardiac insufficiency. Cardiac catheterization is possible now because of the significantly decreased risk associated with the procedure. New catheters used to visualize the coronary arteries result in minimally disruptive procedures that allow patients to go home several hours after the examination. Cardiac catheterization will be a large and growing portion of hospital ambulatory care programs as companies continue to develop less-invasive techniques. The patient population for such procedures is tremendous. According to the National Center for Health Statistics, cardiac catheterizations have been increasing by 100,000 per year since 1984.

Percutaneous Transluminal Coronary Angioplasty

Percutaneous transluminal coronary angioplasty (PTCA), commonly referred to as balloon angioplasty, is an innovative technique that dilates coronary arteries that are affected by coronary plaque in order to restore normal blood flow to damaged heart tissue. Currently, 30 percent of coronary artery bypass surgery patients are candidates for PTCA. Although PTCA is a relatively new procedure, its use is increasing dramatically. No procedures were performed in 1980, approximately 150,000 were done in 1986, and 400,000 are predicted to be done by 1990.[3]

The success rates for PTCA since 1980 have exceeded 80 percent, and the efficacy of this technique in the outpatient setting has been even more astounding. In one study over a six-year period conducted at Presbyterian Hospital in Albuquerque, New Mexico, fewer complications and failures resulted when angioplasty was performed on an outpatient basis than on an inpatient basis. The failure rate was nearly 7 percent for inpatient angioplasties, but only 4 percent for outpatient angioplasties. Although patients undergoing riskier procedures were kept in the hospital, the physicians conducting the study emphasized that outpatient angioplasty is safe and cost-effective. During the study period (1981 to 1987), the use of outpatient angioplasty resulted in savings in hospital-stay costs of $150,000.[4]

Ultra-Fast CT

Technological breakthroughs in noninvasive techniques for the diagnosis of cardiovascular disease, such as Ultra-Fast CT, will be one of the fastest-growing areas in diagnostic imaging. Ultra-Fast CT allows for the direct visualization of heart function through its ability to make stop-action movies of the heart. It can visualize both anatomical and physiological information about the beating heart; for example, it can view the internal chambers and evaluate heart muscle, and in some cases it has been used to evaluate lung and chest masses.

   Clinical studies of Ultra-Fast CT have demonstrated that it is quite effective, and perhaps superior to such other imaging modalities as angiography, nuclear medicine, and echocardiography. In fact, Ultra-Fast CT has been widely documented as providing more specific diagnostic information than magnetic resonance imaging (MRI) in cardiology applications. In the future, Ultra-Fast CT will be scrutinized for its potential in noncardiac procedures. Some proponents predict that Ultra-Fast CT could become so pervasive that it could replace conventional computed tomography (CT). Still others contend that it could replace conventional CT and grow by another 30 to 40 percent through its substitution for such other procedures as angiography, cardiac catheterization, ultrasound, and nuclear medicine procedures.[5] In any event, it may become a major component of diagnostic imaging for ambulatory care environments because it is easily installed and used in the outpatient setting.

Magnetic Resonance Imaging

The 1970s was the decade for the emergence of computed tomography (CT), and although it is still considered the modality of choice for abdominal examinations, magnetic resonance imaging (MRI) is CT's counterpart for the 1980s and beyond. Magnetic resonance imaging is truly one of the most prominent new technologies of this decade; it has brought more progress to diagnostic medicine in the past 15 years than occurred in the entire history of medicine, according to some experts. Unlike conventional X rays, MRI is a combination of radio waves and a strong magnetic field. As such, MRI is superior to other modalities because it can visualize within bone structures and can depict soft tissues in high contrast. It is already showing dramatic improvements over conventional CT in studies of brain visualization, the brain stem, and the cervical spine. As it is enhanced in the future, MRI will eventually be utilized in the entire body.[6] Because of MRI's current potential, it should pass the national distribution of CT procedures by the early 1990s. In addition, MRI's future will be an ambulatory care consideration — it is estimated that as many as 80 percent of MRI procedures will be performed on outpatients in the future.

Ultrasound

Of the various major technologies in the ambulatory care setting, ultrasound has experienced the greatest growth. Its sales now exceed that of any other imaging modality, including MRI and CT. Generally, the acceptance of ultrasound has occurred and expanded because of its relative ease of use, enhanced diagnostic capabilities, and high-quality images. Because of its relatively low cost, ultrasound equipment can pay for itself in less than one year.

Ultrasound utilizes high-frequency sound waves that are transmitted through the surface of the body and reflect echo waves that are electronically decoded to yield important medical information. As such, ultrasound can be used for many clinical studies throughout the body. Primary applications today include radiology, cardiology, vascular imaging, urology, obstetrics and gynecology, and ophthalmology. In addition to these applications, several specialty purposes have emerged in the areas of breast scanning and expanded genitourinary uses.

In the future, ultrasound increasingly will be utilized in diagnosing disturbances of cardiac function and vascular flow that currently are being diagnosed with more expensive technologies. Thus, as developments increase, more overlap will occur with competing technologies. In some instances, current modalities may quickly become obsolete in specified clinical applications. For instance, ultrasound is excellent for examining soft tissue abnormalities in the abdomen, whereas MRI and CT are superior for the neck and head regions, where ultrasound cannot easily penetrate.

MR Spectroscopy

The emergence of MRI and its potential for imaging the entire body has led to the study of anatomical information and its relationship to biochemical functioning, or spectroscopy. Although it is unlikely in the near future that such integration will occur, the long-term impact of this research will be far-reaching. MR spectroscopy may be useful in the assessment of biochemistry and in monitoring the effectiveness of therapeutic interventions in such diseases as cancer. However, its current use emphasizes examination of the brain. Once tumors are located, an analysis of their makeup can easily be obtained. MR spectroscopy, if effective and accepted, will revolutionize the provision of imaging services. Its impact on ambulatory care will be equally dramatic.

Lithotripsy

Extracorporeal shock-wave lithotripsy, commonly referred to as lithotripsy, is a procedure that uses high-energy shock waves to pulverize kidney stones into gravel-like fragments that patients usually pass within several weeks. An investigational procedure in the mid-1980s, it is currently a routine alternative to kidney stone surgery and, more recently, to gallstone surgery as well. It also represents a substantial market; 250,000 kidney stone patients have received lithotripsy in the past three years. Because gallstone surgeries outnumber kidney stone surgeries by a ratio of four to one, the demand for gallstone lithotripsy could be very large.

This technology will continue to evolve, not only in terms of patients treated, but also in the technology utilized. Devices will become more cost-effective, smaller, more efficient, and more versatile. For instance, a new compact, portable kidney stone lithotripter has been developed that eliminates the need for a water bath, can be provided by any conventional X-ray fluoroscopy unit that has a C-arm, and utilizes a conventional operating table or specially designed treatment table. In addition, piezoelectric lithotripsy, which utilizes continuous ultrasound for stone localization and ultrashort pressure waves for kidney stone disintegration, can be performed without anesthesia. The cost of procedures using the piezoelectric device is 40 percent less than traditional lithotripters, because they eliminate the use of fluoroscopy. This technology will greatly affect those institutions that acquire it, because almost all patients needing lithotripsy can be treated as outpatients.

Surgical Laser Technology

Laser technology is increasingly popular as an acquisition and development strategy for many hospitals, initiated primarily because of advances in the equipment utilized and a reduction in their costs. Overall, surgical lasers have the important benefits of lessening recovery time while also decreasing the cost of procedures in comparison with conventional surgical methods.[7] Lasers will have an important role in ambulatory care because they are being used increasingly for outpatient procedures.

Four major surgical laser systems are currently in use: (1) argon laser, used primarily in ophthalmology, plastic surgery, and gastroenterology; (2) carbon dioxide laser, which is used in neurosurgery, otolaryngology, and gynecology; (3) neodymium: yttrium-aluminum-garnet (Nd:YAG), which is available in two forms — one consisting of a continuous wave of light energy, which is used primarily in gastrointestinal applications to seal bleeding vessels and ulcers, and one using pulsed energy or shock waves, which is used in ophthalmic procedures to break apart tissue; and (4) tunable dye laser, which permits the selection of a variety of wavelengths that can be absorbed by different tissues to either coagulate or vaporize the tissue. It is predicted that three out of four hospitals in the United States will have surgical laser technology in use by 1990.[8] This technology will continue to evolve, with future development of new types of lasers and expanded uses for those currently available. Surgical laser technology will create a great challenge for hospitals as more former inpatient surgeries will be done on an outpatient basis using lasers. Although it has been widely reported that approximately 40 percent of total hospital admissions are for surgical cases, nearly 45 percent of surgeries are now outpatient; this figure will increase to 60 percent of all surgeries by 1995.[9]

Endoscopy

New developments in endoscopy have had a great impact on the practice of gastroenterology. Since the introduction of fiberoptic scopes in the 1970s that visualize the entire digestive tract, diagnosis and treatment of digestive disorders have improved tremendously. Growth in this area has been so positive that many institutions now realize that demand for such services exceeds their facility capacity and available resources. This trend will continue as hospitals seek expansion opportunities and as technological advances in this area keep pace with that growth.

One example of a technological advance is the recent introduction of endoscopic ultrasound. This technique is accomplished when conventional endoscopy is utilized in conjunction with ultrasound capabilities to produce high-resolution cross-sectional images of any abnormalities. In other words, the physician can immediately define a lesion as local or diffuse, measure its size, and define how deep it has penetrated and how far it has spread. In another example, fiberoptic endoscopes have been utilized recently to locate chronic gastrointestinal bleeding. In this procedure, a topical anesthetic is used while the enteroscope is inserted along with a pediatric colonoscope. After medication has stimulated passage of the enteroscope, the small portion of the intestinal tract can be viewed. Interestingly enough, this procedure can diagnose gastrointestinal bleeding in 15 minutes on patients for whom angiography or exploratory surgery has failed, and it can be performed on an outpatient basis. Although some institutions consider endoscopy procedures to be separate from outpatient surgery programs, the growth of less-invasive surgery, such as endoscopy, will comprise a large portion of the fundamental shift from inpatient to outpatient surgeries in the future.

Interventional Radiology

The trend toward less-invasive surgery has led to a new technological specialty in radiology services that is often referred to as interventional radiology. Interventional radiology is a process of using new therapeutic tools to treat diseases throughout the body without surgery. Interventional radiologic procedures are unified by the fact that they are performed percutaneously and are monitored and guided by observing an X-ray image of the patient. Specific problems that can utilize interventional catheters include blocked or occluded vessels that can be opened by infusing a particular medication. One example is the alleviation of arterial blockages in patients with leg pain caused by limited blood flow that is depriving tissue of needed oxygen. A number of medical problems increasingly will be treated by nonsurgical techniques developed by interventional radiologists. As technological advances increase, all but a portion of these procedures will be performed in ambulatory settings.

Positron Emission Tomography

Positron emission tomography (PET) is a recent entrant in the field of health care technology. Although it is controversial because of its high cost and complexities to build and operate, it promises tremendous efficacy in the future. Whereas other imaging technologies depict the structure of bones and tissues, PET assesses the biochemical and physiological functioning of such organs as the brain and heart. In general, PET tracks the activity of radioactive, positron-emitting isotopes injected into the body. The system uses computer analysis to generate a three-dimensional image from a series of radiation measurements.

Studies suggest that PET does, in fact, provide valuable information that other technologies do not. For instance, PET can detect metabolic activity in heart muscle that appears dead when imaged by other methods. It has also been found to detect abnormalities in the brain much more precisely than other methods, because it can yield information about whether a tumor is continuing to grow or is responding to treatment. Unfortunately, this technology is still being developed and will require additional research to evaluate its cost and benefit.

The capital cost of PET is quite high because it often requires a cyclotron — a particle accelerator — to make the radioactive isotopes that are required to visualize tissues and organs. Currently these scanners, including cyclotron and installation of equipment, can cost from $2 million to $5 million. Despite the ongoing debate on cost and efficacy, hospitals are beginning to acquire this new technology in order to achieve a strategy of long-term positioning in imaging services.

Single-Photon Emission Computed Tomography

Not to be confused with positron emission tomography (PET), single-photon emission computed tomography, or SPECT, is an imaging modality that provides three-dimensional radionuclide imaging information, estimates regional blood flow, and measures organ volumes. It is essentially a merger of two diagnostic techniques: the gamma camera used in radionuclide imaging and the computerized methods of processing data developed for X-ray transmission computed tomography (CT). Thus, whereas conventional CT provides imaging views one dimension at a time, SPECT acquires many transverse views simultaneously to provide three-dimensional pictures.

Although SPECT has been proven to be two to three times less sensitive than PET, it has several advantages over PET. In cardiovascular applications, SPECT provides continuous data samples of the heart in action from all possible viewpoints, whereas similar reconstructions from PET analysis require frequent repositioning of the patient and the recording of several sets of data. Also, SPECT offers improvements in certain liver and bone imaging applications to make it superior to planar scanning. Perhaps its greatest advantage over PET is one of cost—SPECT systems cost as little as $300,000 compared to $2 million to $5 million for PET.

Because this technology is still evolving, knowledge about its role in diagnostic imaging is incomplete. Considerable research and development will continue, making this a closely monitored application for the future. It could become a highly desired application, because preliminary research indicates that it may accurately measure cerebral blood flow to diagnose impending cerebral infarctions and other brain physiological activity.

Topographic Brain Mapping

Topographic brain mapping (TBM) is a relatively new method utilized to diagnose various kinds of brain pathology, such as tumors, trauma, seizures, and multiple sclerosis. Actually, it is an outgrowth of early technology in electroencephalography (EEG) studies. Instead of displaying multiple traces from EEG equipment, TBM creates a colored map of the scalp. Although EEG tracings are still used, the outcome display is different. Despite controversy regarding its effectiveness, there is some evidence that TBM often can enhance the accuracy of EEG as well as expand the application of EEG to some disorders where previously it has not been very useful. Overall, although no new information is derived from TBM, the findings of TBM are more easily apparent than those of EEG because much of the subjectivity of interpretation of the EEGs is removed. Although computerized tomography and magnetic resonance imaging have been used in place of some previous EEG studies, TBM will likely be used for those functional disorders whose origin cannot be identified. Also, because TBM procedures are noninvasive, they will continue to be important components of hospital ambulatory care environments, particularly for those hospitals that establish comprehensive neurology programs.

Picture Archiving and Communication Systems

The recent trend toward digital image management and transmission associated with diagnostic procedures has led to an industry definition of picture archiving and communication systems, or PACS. Generally, these systems store valuable information taken from images that can then be transmitted via computer terminals to off-site locations. For hospitals, PACS reduce the need to use and store costly X-ray film, enhance the quality of images, achieve cost savings through fewer repeat examinations, and enable transmission to on-call radiologists or back-up specialty consultants.

In the long term, PACS will help reduce patients' lengths of stay by reducing the time needed to process test results. Unfortunately, these systems are still developing, and it will be several years before they are widely accepted. Current costs are prohibitive for most institutions: more than $2 million for some systems. Until PACS are available, hospitals can take advantage of the many teleradiology systems currently in use that allow current and digitalized films to be transmitted via telephone. With these systems, conventional analog films are placed under a video camera, are digitalized via computer, and then are transmitted by telephone. Once the digitalized films are displayed on the receiving monitor, images can be manipulated to enhance contrast. As teleradiology technology further evolves with PACS systems, the potential for regionalization of certain imaging modalities and their professional interpretation will be enormous. This trend will also significantly affect the level, scope, and management of outpatient imaging services.

Laboratory Testing

As discussed elsewhere in this book, advances in laboratory technology and a changing payment system for services are quickly altering the provision of laboratory testing. From an ambulatory care perspective, these advances and changes will enable providers to deliver a wider array of services in a much shorter time period. Automated analyzers, for instance, can improve stat turnaround times, decrease costs, and occupy dedicated areas or remote sites. Perhaps the greatest role in the future of laboratory testing will be played by information systems that can provide rapid turnaround of multiple test results in both hospital-based and freestanding settings. Once integrated with the hospital's information system, these systems can provide unlimited opportunities to access previous medical history and data. This will be an important era for hospitals that provide ambulatory care, because data management availability will also enable physicians to schedule ambulatory tests and procedures at the same time. This convenience factor alone will positively affect the future provision of ambulatory care services.

Objective Technology Planning

Much has been written regarding the assessment and acquisition of medical technology. Unfortunately, although many understand its merits, few have heeded the advice. Regrettably, some technologies are acquired that fail to meet provider expectations, are underutilized, and produce negative operating results. In today's environment, failure to plan adequately for technological change could significantly alter an institution's market positioning. As ambulatory care development and expansion become top priorities, the amount and mix of patient shifting to the outpatient setting will, to a large degree, be a function of the technology selected.

The Commitment to Technology

The commitment to technology involves careful assessment and planning. A critical phase in technology assessment and acquisition for ambulatory care services is the incorporation of technology review as a distinct component of the strategic planning process. Technology review must be part of the institution's mission, goals, and objectives. Failure to ensure this will lead to uninformed decisions, unnecessary duplication of efforts, and potentially disastrous results.

Although many institutions consider ambulatory care technology to be a segment of the entire inpatient technology planning process, it needs to be identified as a separate component. Increasingly, the future of technology will be in the ambulatory setting; current inpatient technologies that become obsolete will be replaced by ambulatory alternatives, prospective payment systems will eventually result in a shifting of ambulatory care technology to office-based and other freestanding environments, and self-diagnostic procedures will become more commonplace in nonhospital environments. Because hospitals are, and will continue to be, focal points of the health care system, they will play a significant role in technology placement.

Market-Based Planning

The assessment and acquisition of ambulatory care technology must be based on a thorough understanding of each institution's local and regional markets. To gain this understanding, specialized advice must be incorporated from the many individuals who participate in the various phases of a technology's utilization. Market-based planning provides information on what the market will support and avoids the difficulty of trying to induce demand for a particular technological service. Thus, a multidisciplinary group that includes, among others, physicians, nurses, and support personnel can appropriately determine specific objectives of a particular technology. This type of planning lessens the potential for an improper direction and decision. Finally, planning for service acquisition must ultimately consider the financial ramifications. If services cannot produce positive financial results in a relatively short time, they must be seriously questioned. The prospective payment system for ambulatory care, whatever its final outcome, will not necessarily reward the acquisition of new technology.

The Operational Impact of Technology

Although a new technology may fill a marketplace need and may be financially viable, its operational impact on other services and similar technology still must be assessed. Such personnel issues as recruitment and training are as important as the acquisition itself. If personnel are not readily available or will be underutilized, staffing and turnover may become significant issues, particularly in small or rural hospital settings. In addition, a series of organizational impact analyses must be performed to evaluate facility installation requirements, support technology modifications, and costs of utilities and installation. Hospitals will find these impact analyses to be particularly difficult; they involve many variables and often result in many trade-offs. It is likely that in the future, technology acquisitions will be limited to those that have a different level of operational impact—those that reduce costs by eliminating procedures, reduce diagnostic times, and enhance the shift to predominantly outpatient environments.

References

1. Matson, T. A. Rethinking the delivery of ambulatory care: hospital-based versus freestanding alternatives. Presentation, Penetrating the Alternate Site Marketplace Conference, Biomedical Business International, Inc., San Francisco, Sept. 15, 1987.

2. Technology scan: emerging diagnostics and therapeutics. *Hospital Strategy Report* 1(3): 7, 1989.

3. Rubin, C. Outpatient cardiac care. *Medicenter Management,* Mar. 1988, p. 22.

4. Outpatient angioplasties deemed safer and more effective. *Medicenter Management,* July 1988, p. 14.

5. Burns, M. Cine-CT: progress and opportunities. *Hospital Technology Series— Guideline Report* 5:20, 1986.

6. Steiner, K. Personal communications. *Siemens AG Bereich Medizinische Technik.* Erlangen, West Germany, 1986.

7. Linn, B. Market memo: hospital use lags behind lasers' tremendous potential. *Health Care Strategic Management* 7(8):1, Aug. 1989.

8. Alder, H. C. Implementing laser technology in the community hospital. *Hospital Technology Series—Guideline Report* 5:9, 1986.

9. Matson.

Chapter 7

Operational Considerations

Theodore A. Matson

Despite the growing importance of ambulatory care services, hospital outpatient departments have received a disproportionately small share of the hospitals' total physical, technical, and medical resources. Consequently, current facility and space requirements for ambulatory care services are inadequate; patients have long waits for procedures and often are a second priority to all inpatients; departments are located within many different areas of the hospital; and the overall provision of services is fragmented.

This second-class status is unfortunate, because the delivery of hospital ambulatory care services is a very complex process. Many patients who use outpatient services are unscheduled, have multiple tests performed in more than one department, and visit a very unfamiliar environment. In short, the typical patient endures a very chaotic experience. Because patients and providers now demand that services be provided in aesthetically pleasing and convenient settings, hospitals must adapt to these demands.

From an operational perspective, a new philosophy must be embraced to effectively meet the demands of ambulatory care services. Programs must be organizationally structured for success and become top priorities for the board of trustees and senior management. To effectively manage the ambulatory care environment, state-of-the-art systems must be in place to monitor and carry out effective decision making in fast-paced situations. Managers will continually face more hands-on operational duties than mere supervision in order to ensure that decisions are executed, monitored, and evaluated rapidly. Overall, health care managers will have to acquire the philosophy and actions of entrepreneurs. They must assume a true business orientation for all profit and loss decisions; act as innovators to continually seek out new and different approaches of managing resources, personnel, and service offerings; acquire an aggressive mentality and political astuteness to defend actions and positions; and exhibit a leadership style that involves and rewards participative team management, yet that recognizes the success of each program or service on an individual basis. Although this will be an extremely difficult period of transition for hospitals and their employees, it nonetheless represents the stark reality of the characteristics that are necessary to compete effectively in the new health care environment.

The advent of a fully prospective payment system will largely determine the structure of the ambulatory care environment in the future. For some hospitals, fixed payments for services will cause a permanent financial loss from operations because of lower patient utilization, amounts and types of patients treated, and facility/organizational structures. At this point, hospitals will have only a few options: (1) continue to operate at a loss, emphasizing a community service orientation; (2) reorganize into a structure that lessens operational loss and provides break-even or marginally profitable status; and (3) discontinue programs or services entirely. A few hospitals can be expected to discontinue some services, particularly those institutions that simply cannot support the necessary utilization and mix of patients required. Therefore, innovation and a strong business and strategic-planning orientation will be required to implement operational changes that ensure the viability of ambulatory services.

An Entrepreneurial Philosophy

As was mentioned earlier, an entrepreneurial philosophy will be essential if hospitals are to compete effectively in the new health care environment. The success or failure of organizations is widely recognized as being dependent on the corporate culture embraced by the chief executive officer and the governing board. Because management philosophy is "top-down," failure to execute proper direction results in a failure to recognize opportunities. Thus, the corporate philosophy will determine the extent to which competitive positioning can be achieved. For hospitals, if ambulatory care is not considered top priority, the long-term viability of ambulatory care programs will be questionable. To achieve the competitive edge in ambulatory services delivery, therefore, the corporate culture of each institution must reflect a commitment to ambulatory care. This will require a redefinition of the hospital's primary mission, goals, and objectives to reflect the specific and unique needs of ambulatory care patients, services, and providers. A long-range strategic plan must be developed exclusively for ambulatory care, and individual business plans must be developed for each service or departmental offering. Realistic goals for projected revenues, market penetration, and financial returns must be developed and continuously monitored.

The ultimate winners in the ambulatory care marketplace will be aggressive and innovative. Unfortunately, the current organizational structure of most hospitals provides disincentives for ambulatory care innovation in comparison with their freestanding counterparts. Each hospital must seek an organizational structure that allows it to create management efficiencies, increase operating flexibility, and enhance the rate of reimbursement. This structure must allow maximum freedom to operate, with appropriate rewards given to those who accept the necessity of risk taking and are successful in their endeavors.

Staffing and patient care delivery in the ambulatory care setting depend largely on the extent to which each institution can become innovative. An innovative philosophy may well become how fewer personnel can be utilized in the provision of patient care; how different types of personnel can be substituted for other personnel alone, or in conjunction with other staff; and how each staff member can be motivated to perform additional tasks not in the domain of his or her normal duties. Although such innovation may be known as a "lean and mean" management philosophy, it is unfortunately an operational reality in the new health care environment.

Finally, successful innovation in ambulatory services delivery must also have as a counterpart a strong consideration for a "back to basics" philosophy. Only programs that clearly demonstrate need, have an adequate patient population for effective program utilization, and can achieve profitability in a short period of time should be implemented. In the previous cost-based environment for ambulatory care services, numerous programs that could not meet these criteria were supported through cross-subsidization by other programs. Now that a fully prospective payment system for ambulatory care is near implementation, this operational philosophy is no longer appropriate. Failure to embrace a true "bottom-line" orientation for services will no doubt result in numerous programs that suffer permanent financial losses. In every respect, service offerings in the future must be tied to the overall goals of the institution. Only those institutions that develop services that specifically fill a market void will be assured of operational success.

Moving toward Operational Efficiency: Getting the Right Data

Achieving managerial efficiency through operations will be a formidable task for many ambulatory care programs. For those institutions that can support it and are committed to it, a full-service integrated ambulatory care facility will solve problems associated with inadequate patient access, scattered departments throughout the hospital, favoring inpatient procedures over outpatient procedures, and the logistical chaos of multiple patients transported to multiple departments. For others, the tasks will be much more complex, yet not beyond the realm of the institution. In all cases, achieving efficiency will largely be dependent upon how operational information is collected and utilized. For the entire system of ambulatory care, information on utilization, productivity, staffing, expenses, payer mix, and financial performance must be collected, analyzed, and strictly adhered to for operational decision making. Not only should this information be prepared in aggregate for ambulatory care, but also at the individual program or "subsystem" level to provide comparative trends against which to evaluate each business plan's projected goals and objectives. Unfortunately, much of these data do not exist in most institutions and must be developed manually. Yet, if ambulatory care programming is to be successful, effective data collection is imperative in order to make appropriate decisions.

In designing a data management analysis system for ambulatory care services, a core set of operational parameters should be collected on a monthly, quarterly, and yearly basis. Each institution may also have specific data needs for unique services or clinics that should be considered as components of this master data strategy. Generally, data reporting should consist of service or procedural utilization by individual procedure or service; procedural revenue by primary source data; staffing expenses by paid hours, worked hours, and salaries by personnel type; and expenses of supplies, equipment, and facility-related costs.

Staffing Data

The clear defining and recording of staffing paid hours, work hours, and salary expenses is critical in the ambulatory care environment. Much of the economies of scale in the outpatient setting will be determined by the extent to which staffing patterns and expenses can be measured, monitored, and modified. Among paid hours, the total accrued hours for which employees are paid, both time spent at work and nonworked time, is also a common reporting requirement. They should be differentiated by the level of each worker: nursing hours; technical hours; clerical hours; administrative/supervisory hours; and hours for other skill levels, such as orderlies, housekeepers, laboratory workers, and radiology personnel. Conversely, worked hours exclude nonworked hours, such as vacation, holiday, and sick days, but are differentiated according to the same classification of skill levels. It is important to carefully define those hours that are contracted from outside labor pools, as ambulatory care services increasingly are being provided by contract management firms. Finally, salary expenses are reported as accrued wages to employees, including amounts paid for vacations, holidays, call-time, and overtime, and are identified under the appropriate skill level classification.

Revenue Data

Recording all gross patient revenue directly attributable to the specific function of each program or service is a uniform data reporting requirement.

In addition, for procedures not provided directly by a department, revenue from these sources should also be clearly identified with the department ordering the service. These data are becoming increasingly important as decisions are made to add services to a particular department or to convert an entire operating unit into a freestanding entity. For instance, although emergency departments do not directly perform a wide variety of procedures and tests, emergency patients comprise significant volumes of tests performed by other departments. It is estimated that 20 to 30 percent of laboratory volume originates in the emergency department, and 40 to 60 percent of outpatient radiology procedures are performed for these patients.[1] Thus, new equipment acquisitions for radiology or laboratory applications may be greatly influenced by the ordering and test requests of the emergency department.

In addition to reporting gross revenues and deductions from revenues as a result of contractual allowances, discounts, personnel adjustments, the provision for bad debts, and so forth, primary payer source revenue must be identified for every patient, and preferably for each individual procedure or service. Medicare, Medicaid, Blue Cross, private insurance, and self-pay are common carriers; HMO, PPO, and managed health care arrangements are not as predominant. It is particularly important to specifically identify these new payers, because some institutions now receive nearly 50 percent of their revenues from contractual arrangements. Collectively, these data will yield uniform reporting of all financial, statistical, and operational parameters, not only for each service, but for the entire ambulatory care environment as well. Although this methodology will benefit operational decision making, it is very time-consuming and costly. To assist in the formulation of data reporting, the following sections provide definitional requirements of the general information to be collected.

Statistical Data

It is imperative to collect and report statistical data on all utilization associated with each ambulatory care service or procedure. For instance, ambulatory surgery may be differentiated not only according to the overall number of patients treated, but also by the specific type and range of services or procedures performed. For each procedure, the type of anesthesia utilized — general, regional, local, monitored, or none — should be identified. Emergency department patients should be listed not only by the total number of patients treated, but by the number of patients per time of day, by those resulting in an inpatient admission, discharge, or transfer, and by the type of visit — medical, trauma, burn, psychiatric, and so forth. In essence, the more data that can be collected, the more sensitive the specific patient profiles that can be developed.

Expense Data

Expense data is a routine reporting requirement, yet it is important to scrutinize the accrual of expenses incurred to the appropriate expense categories. These include expenses for medical and office supplies, medical equipment and rentals, office equipment depreciation/rentals, and such other direct expenses as laboratory and radiology nonsalary costs, consultant fees, equipment maintenance contracts, marketing costs, laundry and linen costs, educational costs, and recruitment costs. This attention to detail will be valuable when specific profiles of expense categories are evaluated in relation to other ambulatory care functions.

Other Useful Data

Once the uniform reporting of statistical, financial, and operational data is accomplished, a variety of ongoing evaluations of service performance can be developed. Although the previously described data parameters are now standard in many institutions, other information, such as data on operational changes from specific time periods (relative to internal standards and external comparison groupings), will raise many questions regarding real versus perceived operating performance. For instance, trend data for a specific time period may indicate that (1) patient utilization in the emergency department has been declining; (2) nursing and technical salary expenses have increased substantially; and (3) payer mix information yields essentially flat revenues over previous reporting periods. In addition, because of a perceived increase in the acuity of seriously ill patients and frequent complaints of long waiting times by patients, nursing staff have requested additional personnel. Although comparative reporting of data does indicate several interesting operational changes, not enough is known regarding whether the perception of a higher case mix is correct. This situation, therefore, requires that further analysis be conducted to confirm whether there is an increase in the case mix and, if so, whether additional staffing is required or whether a redistribution or mix of personnel is necessary.

The Operational Audit

Auditing of specific operational characteristics in the ambulatory care setting is imperative to determine the level and extent of necessary changes. If quantitative analyses are not performed, current problems might be worsened through misdirected efforts. The operational audit of departmental or service performance can be conducted by numerous methods; however, a simple and practical methodology will include certain criteria. Similar to the data elements involved in the uniform reporting described previously, the operational analysis should consist of data on departmental utilization according to:

1. Visit or procedure by time of day and day of week
2. Duration of patient encounter and/or procedure
3. Zip code origin of residence and employer (if related to workers' compensation)
4. Age and sex of patient
5. Nature of visit—convenience, routine, urgent, or emergency
6. Patient status—new patient, established patient with new episode, or established patient with same problem (series patient)
7. Primary payer source
8. Primary payment mode—Medicare, Medicaid, self-pay, commercial insurance, currency, check, or multiple payers
9. Payment amount or disposition
10. Charges incurred and type—as professional component, ancillaries, medications, and supplies
11. Disposition of patient—home, return to work, physician referral, or other
12. Follow-up care—none, physician referral, medical rehabilitation, or scheduled visit
13. Patient's physicians, including referring physicians and consultants

With a minimum data set to collect, additional information may be incorporated according to the specific needs of each study. Although some data may seem irrelevant to some operational reviews, they should be collected to determine baseline data and the likelihood of future analysis.

Once the parameters are determined, a review of the operation can be performed utilizing a simple chart-auditing methodology. Thus, a simple random sampling of every fifth or tenth chart during a specific time interval and a patient population of 200 to 300 usually will yield valid interpretations. Generally, auditing via a single hard copy form will be sufficient for initial data collection prior to data input and analysis. Once this information is stored in a data base management program, an infinite series of operational profiles of departmental performance can be obtained. At this point, management must decide what actions can be instituted solely on the merits of the data. In many situations, the eventual outcomes will lead to easily understood problems and solutions; however, in some instances a more quantitative and broad-based study will be necessary. This latter approach will require an extensive and focused operational review of the department or service in question, concentrating primarily on parameters of interdepartmental relationships, fluctuations in work-load volume, scheduling, mix of personnel involved, and staffing patterns. Although this methodological approach may be warranted, it is often costly to execute and should be used only when simplified methods do not suffice.

Financial Management and Reimbursement

Operational success in providing ambulatory care services will also depend to a large degree on how and whether payment policies provide incentives for efficient delivery and utilization of services. Until recently, Medicare payment for all hospital outpatient services was based on cost-reimbursement principles. Today, payment for a single outpatient encounter may now involve four different payment methodologies: (1) fee-for-service payment for clinical laboratory services; (2) a blended prospective payment rate for certain outpatient surgical services; (3) blended prospective payment rate for outpatient radiology procedures; and (4) reasonable cost for all other hospital outpatient services.

With recent legislation mandating a fully prospective payment system for all ambulatory care services by 1991, Medicare will be the first payer to develop a capitated system of payment. Once this system is implemented, a number of other major payers are expected to endorse a similar approach to outpatient payment. In fact, some managed health care firms are already contracting with hospitals solely on the basis of Current Procedural Terminology (CPT-4) coding for ambulatory surgery payment. Unfortunately, little is known of the eventual framework of a patient classification system for outpatient payment; the current systems are only temporary.

Of the various payment approaches that could be utilized, the Health Care Financing Administration (HCFA) has focused on a system that is based on a fixed fee for providing a package of bundled services. Similar to the intent of the inpatient prospective payment system, incentives would also be created for outpatient payment based on all-inclusive rates that will: (1) reflect a single price for each service regardless of the facility setting; (2) reflect payment rates based on the types of service(s) provided; (3) facilitate monitoring for claims review and auditing purposes; (4) minimize the number of services through prudent service delivery; and (5) control Medicare program growth. Under this classification system, the focus of payment is on the patient visit rather than on the episode of illness. Thus, a system oriented toward paying for bundles of services, rather than individual procedures, will require accurate and reliable coding and abstracting of medical records data to group patients with similar resource consumption.

Regardless of the patient classification system chosen, a number of steps should be implemented to ensure short-term and long-term reimbursement of services provided. Of the partially prospective payment systems that exist currently, ambulatory surgery is the best example to illustrate the demands of code-based reimbursement and record management practices. Since October 1, 1987, fees for hospital outpatient departments performing procedures for ambulatory surgical centers are determined in part according to the prospective payment methodology now used for ambulatory surgery centers. To receive reimbursement, hospitals must use HCFA's Common

Procedural Coding System (HCPCS) for reporting outpatient services. The HCPCS is primarily used by Medicare Part B carriers and Medicaid agencies to determine payment on physician supplier claims. Another system, CPT-4 is a listing of descriptive terms and identifying codes for reporting medical services and procedures performed by physicians. The HCPCS encompasses CPT-4 and includes additional codes for various medical supplies and services that are not provided by physicians and for which CPT-4 codes do not exist.

Hospitals must report HCPCS codes for all significant surgical procedures. Significant surgery is defined as incision, excision, amputation, introduction, repair, destruction, endoscopy, suture, or manipulation. Because of this definition, procedures performed in the emergency department, medical endoscopy suites, or specialty clinics are subject to HCPCS coding for reimbursement. Although hospitals previously reported surgical procedures using the ICD-9-CM procedure coding structure, HCPCS and ICD-9-CM cannot be compared because of the differences in their coding descriptions. Because the addition of CPT-4 surgical codes often exceeds the available space in a hospital's master list of charges, the codable procedures must be added manually to the charge area of the Uniform Bill (UB-82). In addition, charge master records identify surgical utilization according to time units for the use of operating suites; HCPCS must be coded from narrative information sheets or other hospital records.

In essence, the requirements imposed for reimbursement of ambulatory surgical services mean that hospitals will have to maintain two coding systems. Although their freestanding counterparts have always utilized CPT-4 coding as the basis of reimbursement, it is a new phenomenon for hospitals. The ICD-9-CM system will play a large role also, because it will continue to be required by Medicare and other payers. Clearly, this fragmented approach complicates hospital billing, medical record, and accounting procedures. To ensure that reimbursement is maximized, hospitals must adapt by developing new philosophies toward outpatient service management.

Centralized Review of Patient Accounts Management

The logistical and operational chaos that often accompanies outpatient service delivery mandates a coordinated, systematic review of all billing and patient accounts management. Often, many of the problems encountered in the outpatient setting are the result of poor communication between various departments, unnecessary overlap of specific functions, and lack of administrative accountability in the monitoring and problem resolution of certain functions. For instance, billing problems and claim rejections often occur when outpatient registration personnel are inconsistent in ascertaining the exact information required. Generally, this is a result of lack of training or lack of understanding of what information is absolutely necessary.

A monthly operational task force can analyze outpatient registration errors and identify practical resolutions. Because the phasing in of a fully prospective payment system for ambulatory care is nearing, the operational task force can begin to monitor proposed operational requirements. Careful adherence to necessary changes will result in avoiding misdirected efforts after phase-ins begin.

Ensuring Accurate HCPCS/CPT-4 Coding

Traditionally, outpatient coding in most hospitals has been centralized in the business office. Because experience with CPT-4 coding was developed in this area, hospital management has not been concerned with moving the function. However, now that coding is becoming increasingly complex and has a tremendous impact on reimbursement, it is imperative that it be performed by someone with access to the entire medical record. Thus, it is highly desirable to concentrate this function in the medical records department. This strategy is important for several reasons:

- The assignment of codes is highly clinical in nature and subject to much interpretation; medical records personnel are specifically trained in medical interpretation, code selection, and code sequencing, which are critical for accurate HCPCS/CPT-4 coding.
- Outpatient procedures are now taking place in a number of settings; if coding is concentrated in the medical records department, records can be routed more systematically to the persons responsible for CPT-4 coding to ensure coding compliance.
- Medical records personnel's inpatient record-keeping function already links them with medical staff members, so good channels of communication for obtaining attestations, clarification, and documentation necessary for proper coding of outpatient procedures are already established.
- Without the burden of assigning codes, personnel in the business office can concentrate on updating the charge master files to validate that revenue codes that are used for billing are correctly linked to the HCPCS/CPT-4 codes.

Overall, coding is and will continue to be a tremendous challenge for hospitals; a specialized structure with clinical and financial experts will be necessary to maximize Medicare reimbursement.

Superbills and Credit Cards

Aside from preparing for changes dictated by an outpatient payment system for ambulatory care services and by payers that adopt a Medicare-like system for reimbursement, efforts should also focus on innovative strategies that will maximize reimbursement for non-Medicare patients. The ambulatory care environment presents a unique opportunity for such innovation, as patients increasingly want to pay their bills at time of service. One approach receiving wide consumer acceptance is the use of a "superbill" that includes a series of commonly utilized services, such as emergency department, routine laboratory, radiology, and so forth. This listing of tests and procedures can be contained in the hospital's information systems or, preferably, on a single charge master itemization that the patient takes from department to department. Superbills combined with the acceptance of credit cards are a source of fast reimbursement. This is a great improvement in collections, because the average charge for outpatient services is less than $200 per patient, and numerous billings often are sent to a significant number of outpatients in comparison to inpatients.

Historically, hospitals that have accepted credit cards have found that they were underutilized primarily because patients were not aware that hospitals accepted them. For credit cards to be effective, their use must be aggressively promoted through a request for credit card information at the point of registration and through display signs acknowledging the use of credit cards. Although some patient account managers may be leery of using the cards because of such unknowns as a patient's deductible, whether there are multiple insurers, and so forth, there are ways to use the cards advantageously. One way to avoid problems with credit cards is to estimate a patient's bill, charge it to the appropriate card, and then adjust it later if necessary. Overall, hospitals have had good experiences with credit card usage and often find that patients are more willing to pay in full by credit card than by cash or check.

Self-Pay Patients, Debt Collection, and Medicaid Application Assistance

In recent years, there has been a dramatic increase in the number of self-pay and uninsured patients in ambulatory settings. Yet a large portion of charges incurred by these patients is often written off as bad debt. Many account managers have indicated that the dollar figures involved are generally too small in relation to the cost of staff time for efforts at collecting to be beneficial. Although this may be true in some settings, a number of institutions have witnessed enough of an increase in self-pay populations that they warrant attention. Particularly in some emergency departments, the proportion of self-pay patients has risen from 10 to 20 percent to as high as 40 to 50 percent of total emergency department patients. In addition, many patients today have higher than normal return visit rates and higher rates of admission.

The financial problems posed by patients who do not pay their bills have led hospitals to realize that one solution is to help patients gain Medicaid assistance. The ambulatory care environment, by its very nature, provides a significant amount of primary and ambulatory care to patients who are on medical assistance programs or are eligible for Medicaid. Although it is arguable that some patients may not have an incentive to pay their hospital bill, Medicaid or other state assistance enables them to receive other social program benefits. For smaller institutions, in-house staff may have adequate time and expertise to assist patients; larger institutions may find that contracting with a third party is the most cost-effective approach.

Information Systems to Support Operations

Although hospitals have large volumes of ambulatory care data, much of it has to be manually collected and manipulated for operational decision making. Unfortunately, information system vendors have concentrated on inpatient systems and the various reporting requirements associated with the prospective payment system and have neglected ambulatory care data needs. Many vendors consider outpatient services to be simply components of an existing inpatient system and therefore are reluctant to spend significant monies to improve capabilities. In addition, uncertainty about the potential of various schemes for a fully prospective payment system for ambulatory care makes system design difficult. The federal government also is struggling to determine what elements should comprise uniform collection and reporting of ambulatory care data. Until these issues are resolved, an integrated clinical and financial data base for all outpatient programs is highly unlikely.

As products are developed for the ambulatory care environment, a number of its unique needs will emerge. The information systems of the 1990s will no doubt focus on commonly defined measures of ambulatory care units of service; allow timely access to data on patient treatment and centralized patient information; comprise multientry, multilocation, and multiuser capabilities to facilitate decentralized decision making; and incorporate methods for the review of health care resource utilization by specified user-defined reporting requirements. Unfortunately, until these systems are available to meet marketplace needs, solutions will be short-term and rather expensive to create.

Hospitals, therefore, must develop in-house systems or seek modifications to existing software applications. Because each institution is vastly different in the numbers and types of ambulatory programs, customization is often required to attain specific objectives of an information system. Although a number of major vendors do have departmental-specific software systems, these systems often are developed utilizing proprietary operating systems. This creates a very difficult interfacing situation when multiple vendors are involved. Often, hospitals that have acquired many of these decentralized systems simply find them unworkable when they attempt to create an integrated system. Until the use of sophisticated data increases, the refinement of information systems for ambulatory care probably will not occur.

Reference

1. Matson, T. A. The hospital emergency department in transition. Presentation, American Hospital Association Conference, Chicago, July 15, 1986.

Chapter 8

Implications of Managed Care for Ambulatory Care Managers

Richard B. Donker

Despite rapid advances in medical technology, the litigious nature of patients, the nursing shortage, the "graying of America," the threatened "physician glut," AIDS, and every other development that we can find to blame for decreasing operating margins in health care, the most dramatic change in medicine in this century may well be the advent of managed care. Whereas California, Minnesota, and Florida have been, for different reasons, inundated with managed care products for several years, other states are only beginning to see these changes in reimbursement.

The essence of managed care is the organization of unit-based care so that specific patient outcomes can be achieved within fiscally responsible time frames (lengths of stay) while utilizing resources appropriate (in amount and sequence) to the specific case type and the individual patient. The term *unit* refers to the geographic area in which the patient receives care. Units may include areas such as inpatient or ambulatory units or the emergency department. Managed care can be implemented in any nursing care delivery system (for example, primary, team, or functional).[1]

The concept of managed care is poorly understood by many health care managers, particularly in areas that have not been conducive as yet to the development of managed care products. This is unfortunate, because the health care managers who will be the most affected by managed care—the managers of ambulatory care programs—are the very people who can assist hospital executives most in the process of planning and implementing changes that will allow a hospital to cope with managed care.

This chapter provides some basic information for ambulatory care managers both in the clinical and in the financial/administrative areas. Included will be historical background, the influence of alternative delivery systems of reimbursement on alternative delivery systems of care, and tips on contract strategy with emphasis on ambulatory care. There will be heavy emphasis on the history and development of U.S. health care financing, as that seems to be the perspective that best allows an understanding of the present systems.

Background

The history of health care financing in the United States is a fascinating and complex topic to which many articles and books have been devoted. Understanding the genesis of alternative delivery systems (ADS), though, requires only a cursory review of this topic.

The concept of health insurance was not widespread until the 1930s. (Ironically, it was at about this time that the first "alternative delivery system"—the HMO—was introduced on a small scale.) Health insurance evolved primarily as a fee-for-service system, called *indemnity* insurance. This meant that an insurance company would use highly trained statisticians, called actuaries, who were licensed to predict utilization. (To this day, insurance companies and their actuaries are required to be licensed in order to protect citizens who purchase any kind of insurance from losing coverage because of insurance company insolvency. There are other requirements, such as reserve funding in case of catastrophic claims, and so on.) The insurance company would predict the cost of care, based on the predicted services and prices, add administrative and overhead costs, add a profit margin, and divide the total by the number of subscribers. This amount became the insurance *premium,* which the insured paid on a monthly or yearly basis. The insured patient would go to his or her choice of physician, hospital, or other covered provider, pay a *deductible* or *copayment* amount or both, and receive treatment. The patient or the provider then submitted the bill to the insurance company, which then paid the bill (minus the copayment or deductible or both). The bill was paid on a fee-for-service basis—that is, the more that was done to the patient, the more money that was paid out, as long as the service was covered. This type of insurance still exists, and is alive and well in automobile and home insurance and in other types of insurance markets. Very little of this indemnity insurance is left in the health care market, however.[2]

The U.S. government did not really begin to cover the cost of the general population's health care until the 1960s. The federal Medicare program, which provided health insurance benefits primarily to persons over age 65, and the state-administered Medicaid program, which provided health care benefits to the indigent and medically indigent persons, were both established by amendments to the 1965 Social Security Act. When Medicare and Medicaid began, they paid on a "cost-plus," fee-for-service basis just as other health insurance did, except that they disallowed many hospital and physician charges. Government payment made on a cost basis enabled hospitals to live with increased costs, which was the real genesis of the boom in development and acquisition of medical technology. Knowing that some charges would be disallowed or would be subject to deductibles, Medicare recipients who could afford it (and therefore were likely to be pursued for the portion of a bill that Medicare would not pay—the deductible and copayment) purchased a fee-for-service, indemnity insurance policy to cover the balance of any such physician or hospital bill. This particular form of insurance is called "Medicare Supplement" or "Medigap" insurance.

The Move Away from Indemnity Plans

Significant movement away from indemnity-based plans began in the Reagan years, in part due to that administration's policies, but largely due to a general public revolt against the perceived excesses of the medical system—depersonalized overreliance on technology, overpaid practitioners and providers, and the resultant increases in the cost of health care that were making the cost of insurance prohibitive to the working public. Many familiar phrases about health care costs were born during this period—"skyrocketing costs," "rapidly spiraling inflationary costs," "out-of-control cost increases," and so on. Indeed, the cost of health care had risen as a percentage of the gross national product (GNP) from 5.9 percent in 1965 to 10.2 percent in 1982.[3] Not only was the private citizen concerned, but so were private employers and the government, who saw this increasing percentage of their expenses going to purchase health care.

Perhaps coincidentally, both government and private payer groups began to take action almost simultaneously. Private payers began to take advantage of systems that were very similar to those that they had used to buy other products or services—a discount in return for guaranteed volume, or a flat price per "unit." The "unit," in this case, was a day's stay in the hospital, a particular procedure, a patient stay, or even an enrolled employee's health care for an entire year. These programs or systems had various forms and various amounts of risk for the providers.

In searching for ways to control health care costs, providers and payers looked at systems that were previously used. A very early type of plan in the 1970s actually required that the providers at risk be licensed as a type of insurance company. These plans offered care for a person for a set period of time (usually for a year) for a set price. In return, the employee who enrolled in such a plan or the person who purchased such a plan agreed not to go to any other provider except in a true emergency or other stringently controlled circumstances. Because the money went directly to the provider, who took the risk, instead of to a separate "third-party" insurance company, the effect was to combine a health provider network with an insurance company to form a new system that avoided the middleman. This arrangement was called the health maintenance organization, or HMO, because the provider got paid whether or not the patient was seen or treated during the year, so the clear incentive to the provider was to keep the enrollee/ subscriber/patient healthy and out of the doctor's office or hospital.

Health maintenance organizations were carefully regulated by the federal government, and most HMOs sought to be designated "federally qualified" to provide care. The government set the usual standards required of any insurance company, but, in addition, set requirements that would ensure that HMOs did not gain an advantage over other insurance plans by serving only a certain healthy population to the exclusion of the rest. These requirements included certain types of actuarial studies (called "area ratings") that, when combined with requirements to include certain sizes and types of patient populations, opened HMOs to large numbers of people.

The Emergence of Payment Systems

The simplest of payment systems were those in which the payer (self-insured company, union trust fund, or insurance company) asked for a percentage discount from "usual, customary and reasonable" (UCR) charges in return for an assurance that the employees or subscribers would be given incentives to go (be "channeled") to the provider who agreed to this arrangement. As managed care plans evolved, per day (per diem), per case, per procedure, and other payment arrangements were tried. Of course, this entailed increasing risk to the provider.

This began to tread on the legislation that required that companies that are at risk for prepaid services be licensed as insurance companies, use qualified actuaries, and have all of those safeguards that were described for the standard indemnity plan. Feeling understandably sympathetic to the private payer in this regard, though, many state governments passed enabling legislation in the mid-1980s that paved the way for a new form of managed care plan, the preferred provider organization (PPO), with certain restrictions and limitations on the amount of risk that could be taken by the provider without its actually becoming licensed as both an insurance company and as a health care provider. These groups were now free, in these states, to explore many new arrangements, such as exclusive agreements with providers (exclusive provider organizations, or EPOs), joint ventures between insurance companies and provider networks (insured product options, or IPOs), and combinations of fee-for-service plans with small amounts of risk in the form of "withholds" that were paid only if the insurance plan made money, called "managed premium preferred provider organizations" (or M3POs). Small wonder that very quickly these products became known as the "Alphabet Soup"!

Because there were many excess hospital beds and the beginnings of a physician surplus in the early 1980s, preferred provider organizations and their various "alphabet soup" siblings rapidly became more popular and widespread by the mid-1980s. The PPO that evolved operated in many innovative ways (figure 8-1).

It was not until the late 1980s that HMOs began to make a comeback, due in part to an HMO look-alike called a "competitive medical plan," or CMP. Because of the potential for attacking the real cause of health care costs—the demand for service—some states, such as California, passed enabling legislation for CMPs that made the HMO-type plan more viable and attractive. This variation on the HMO retains the same structure and incentives as the HMO, but with the ability to estimate the projected health care utilization of a company or payer population. One unplanned outcome of this legislation is that it allows the CMP to pick healthier groups and more predictable groups, both of which allow less risk and therefore lower premiums. This has created a problem, though, in that other indemnity and managed care programs are left with an increasingly unhealthy client base.

Utilization Review and Managed Care

The attraction of the HMO and CMP to payers was the incentive to control utilization. The control of demand or utilization, if properly performed, should have far better success at controlling health care cost than simply discounting fees. This was the incentive that had led to the formation of the first HMO way back in 1930. As a result of this basic, fundamental realization, all ADS products (HMOs, CMPs, PPOs, and so forth) quickly embraced an element of the HMO that was crucial to its success—utilization review (UR). *Utilization review* is, quite simply, what its name implies—the constant review of care to make sure that it is necessary and appropriate. (Because of the nature of this review, the department that conducts UR often also conducts quality assurance (QA)—hence the "UR/QA" department.) Utilization review includes checks to see if the patient really needs hospitalization (preadmission certification), if surgery needs to be done (second surgical opinion), if other treatment is being performed correctly (concurrent review), and how quickly the patient can be discharged or transferred to a less-expensive setting (discharge planning). Utilization review has become so central to the management of patient cost control that recently even some of the last remaining indemnity programs are using it to create a new form of plan called "managed fee-for-service." In this scenario, the patient still pays premiums and has freedom of choice for provider, but must adhere to strict UR or pay penalties.

Utilization review, or the "management" of patient care, has become the common thread that links all of the health care payment systems that have been discussed—and to a lesser degree—the old, standard, fee-for-service indemnity plan. It is for that reason that all of these "new" types of reimbursement mechanisms that a few years ago were lumped together as "alternative delivery systems" are now commonly called "managed care."

Figure 8-1. Structure of Preferred Provider Organizations

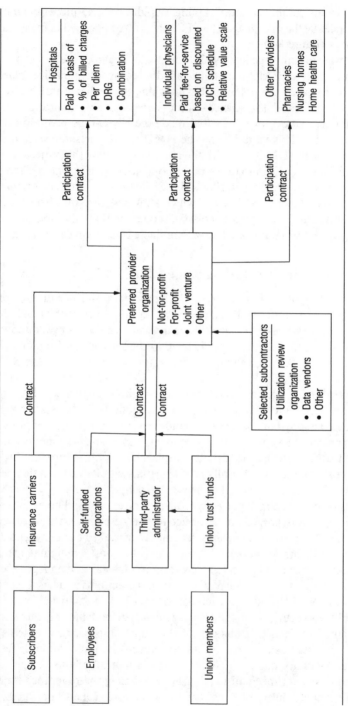

Source: Reprinted from *The PPO Handbook*, by S. B. Barger, D. G. Hillman, and H. R. Garland, p. 5, with permission of Aspen Publishers, Inc., © 1985.

Also of note in this name change is that these systems—HMOs, CMPs, PPOs, EPOs, and so forth—are now, in toto, the standard, not the alternative, as will be shown in the next section.

The Government and Reimbursement

A quick note about the government side of reimbursement is of value here. The government at various levels has taken tacks very similar to those taken by the private sector. At the federal level, Medicare developed the system of diagnosis-related groups (DRGs). Under this system, which currently affects only hospital inpatients (outpatient and physician treatment are still being paid on a cost-based, fee-for-service basis), patients are assigned to one of 477 DRGs. These DRGs are paid at a flat fee, regardless of length or intensity of treatment. There are a few caveats to that, of course, but in effect the government pays on a per-diagnosis or per-case basis, much like a cross between an HMO and a PPO. In addition, Medicare patients have been offered managed care alternatives to their private "Medigap" policies—Medicare PPOs and Medicare HMOs. In these cases, Medicare patients can go only to certain preferred Medicare providers, who treat them in much the same way as private HMO or PPO patients. The discount in this case usually consists of a waiver of all or part of the deductible, copayment or both for Medicare. The federal government also copied the private sector when it recently contracted on a PPO basis for all its Civilian Health and Medical Program of the Uniform Services (CHAMPUS) business on a pilot basis in parts of the western United States.

State governments have also used these methods to control costs. California was among the first and certainly among the most notorious when, in the early 1980s, it named a "MediCal czar" ("MediCal" is California's name for Medicaid), who awarded MediCal service contracts in California to the lowest-priced "bidding" hospitals—a form of the EPO. It further cut costs by removing large blocks of the "working poor" from the MediCal ranks and giving counties a set amount per "medically indigent adult" (MIA) per year—in effect a forced HMO arrangement by virtue of the "capitation," or fixed amount per patient per year.

Virtually all of this has occurred within the past decade. As U.S. health care moves into the 1990s, these systems have had time to mature and solidify. Their effects on the nature and quality of care will continue to have much to do with the delivery of ambulatory care.

How Managed Care and Ambulatory Care Affect Each Other

Managed care formerly was referred to as an "alternative delivery system" with respect to reimbursement. Similarly, ambulatory care is now the term used for the lion's share of those industry reactions to managed care that were termed "alternative delivery systems" of care. This is very confusing, but serves to illustrate the progression of these connections. First, it is important to look at the scope, and projected scope, of managed care. Table 8-1 shows projections for conversions to managed care that were made by experts back in 1986. So far, these estimates have proved to be quite close. Fee-for-service (FFS) medicine is virtually evaporating as indemnity plans are converted to managed FFS or PPO plans. Government plans have always been managed to a certain extent, by virtue of contract provisions and limits on payments, but Medicare PPOs and HMOs have been emerging rapidly since 1987. Clearly, this trend toward managed care is not reversing.

As managed care continues to serve as the primary source of health care reimbursement, the incentives to providers that this care produces will cause further changes in the way in which health care is delivered. These incentives can be easily understood. Fee-for-service or even discounted FFS pays more as more is done for the patient. Figure 8-2 shows that the incentive in these plans has been to increase the number of patients, the length of time that they spend in the hospital, and the procedures (ancillary charges) performed on them while in the hospital. On a per-diem plan, the hospital benefits by having more patients and long stays, but wants the cost per day (per diem) to be low, because payment is a fixed amount per day. In a per-case or per-diagnosis plan (or in the case of a Medicare patient on a DRG), the hospital benefits from more volume (patients), but wants the patient to leave as quickly and inexpensively as possible, because the hospital will receive a fixed amount for the patient's hospital stay, regardless of how long or expensive the treatment.

The ultimate in managed care disincentives to hospitals (and capitated physicians) is the HMO or CMP, which capitates the rates. In this scenario, the physician or hospital is paid a fixed amount per enrollee (not per patient seen) per year. Thus, the provider is best served financially if the enrollee never gets sick, is never seen, and certainly is not hospitalized. Because the provider's incentive is to reduce the amount and types of services provided,

Table 8-1. Estimates for Conversions to Managed Care, 1985–1990

	Private		Government (for those aged 65+)	
	1985	1990	1985	1990
Fee-for-service	77%	15%	0%	0%
Managed-fee-for-service	10	20	96	78
PPO	4	45	0	10
HMO	9	20	4	12

Source: Ernst & Young (formerly Ernst & Whinney), 1986.

Figure 8-2. Incentives to Hospitals under Different Managed Care Models

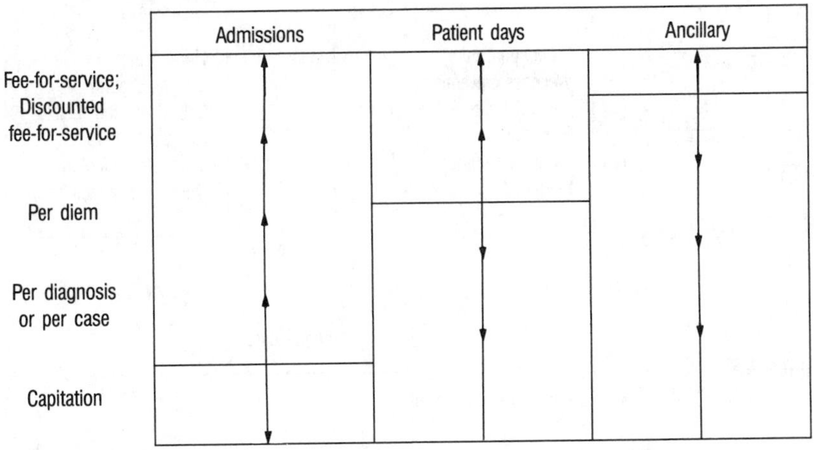

	Admissions	Patient days	Ancillary
Fee-for-service; Discounted fee-for-service			
Per diem			
Per diagnosis or per case			
Capitation			

Source: Memorial Hospitals Association, Inc., 1989.

this can be a perverse incentive. On the other hand, the provider does have an incentive to provide education, screenings, and other preventive measures to help keep the enrollees from becoming ill, and to develop innovative ways to treat patients effectively but less expensively. Effective treatment is presumably ensured, because ineffective treatment would likely involve readmission or at least much more outpatient care, and therefore cost the provider more in the long term.

Providers of health care have, indeed, responded to these incentives. Figure 8-3 shows the relative availability of acute and outpatient or lower-level care. Until the past decade, such things as "wellness programs," "outpatient oncology centers," "freestanding urgent care centers," and "pain clinics" were almost unheard of. Now, these and the other representative types of delivery systems shown in the diagram are commonplace. In order to keep patients from entering the expensive acute inpatient ward (expensive now not only to the payer but to the provider as well), same-day surgery centers are built on a freestanding or less-expensive campus site. Diagnostic centers replace the need for many routine hospital admissions that occur to determine a certain diagnosis or the need for exploratory surgeries. Also, effective prehospital care (paramedic ambulances and helicopters) has been found not only to provide a referral source and a measure of prestige to the sponsoring facility, but also to reduce mortality and morbidity.

Of course, patients will continue to need hospitalization—for trauma and acute infection in the case of the young, and for chronic illnesses in

Figure 8-3. Health Care Provider Responses to Managed Care Incentives

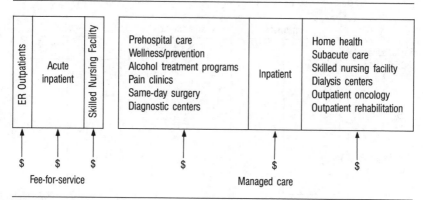

Source: Memorial Hospitals Association, Inc., 1989.

the case of the elderly. The challenge, then, is to transfer the patient as quickly as possible from the acute inpatient facility to an alternative system of care. Home health and rehabilitation centers are such alternatives. The end result, as figure 8-3 illustrates, is that the typical hospital is adding or converting much more space to these alternative systems (most of which are ambulatory care centers) than to acute inpatient beds, resulting in a lower percentage of inpatient space on the campus.

Although, admittedly, some of these "alternative" systems have emerged for other reasons (availability of technology, marketing effectiveness, and so forth), it can be argued that their continued success has frequently been due to managed care. Managed care has helped to create or sustain many of the ambulatory care systems that exist today.

Conversely, these alternative delivery systems have helped to fuel the success of managed care. Without alternatives to acute inpatient care, managed care plans would have plateaued quickly and stagnated as they reached the limits of the traditional hospital's ability to cut costs without obviously endangering the quality of care. This symbiosis of alternative care delivery and alternative financing (managed care) is illustrated by figure 8-4, which compares referral mechanisms under a fee-for-service plan with referral mechanisms ("channeling") under managed care. Under fee-for-service medicine, the patient had no alternative but to see the physician, who referred the patient to the hospital of the physician's choice. With managed care and alternative delivery systems, both the patient and the payer have more decision-making ability. The patient does not require a referral from a physician to visit an urgent care center or pain clinic. The ultimate decision maker, however, is now the third-party payer, who can direct both the patient and

Figure 8-4. Patient Referral Mechanisms: How Alternative Delivery Systems of Financing (Managed Care) Help Create Alternative Delivery Systems of Care (Such As Ambulatory Care)

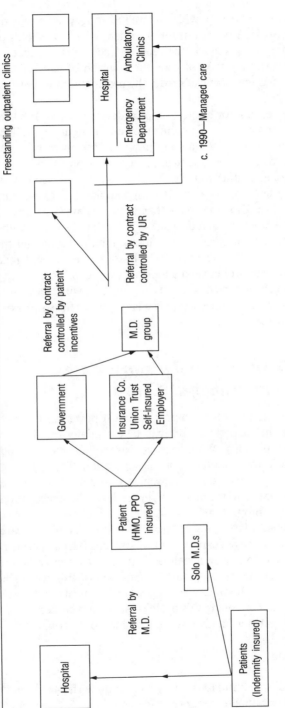

Source: Memorial Hospitals Association, Inc., 1989.

physician to a preferred provider, as well as to a specific type of provider. This is done, of course, by utilization review, which withholds payment to both provider and patient if the preferred choice is not made. Thus, the payer can control the type of care, the location of care, and the amount of care—to an extent that can render the provider almost powerless against the payer.

The only option for health care providers in the past has been to avoid managed care contracts, which some providers have done with limited short-term success. As the battle among providers for an ever-decreasing share of indemnity patients has escalated, though, these providers have been forced by lack of volume either to try to break into the managed care market late or to reduce their scope of care. (It must be pointed out here that the opposite extreme has also occurred—that providers were so anxious to join managed care programs that they did so indiscriminately and without proper cost accounting, resulting in massive losses, unbearable administrative costs, and, in some cases, financial ruin.) The lessons here are clear: managed care is a force that is unavoidable in almost all aspects of health care, participation in managed care must be done carefully and with a strategic plan, and ambulatory care capabilities will play a large part in the success of the hospital in this endeavor.

The Role of the Ambulatory Care Manager in Managed Care

Earlier, it was said that the provider is almost powerless against the payer. This is somewhat hyperbolic, but can be essentially true in a competitive health care community. What leverage can the hospital use, and how is it derived? The answer, quite simply, is reputation. Reputation, in turn, is gained by offering high quality, convenience, and reasonable price, all effectively communicated to the public (or, in marketing language, "product, price, packaging, and promotion").

To this end, a large part of the role of the ambulatory care manager with respect to managed care is to apply strategic business principles. Thus, formulating and following a standard business plan must become regular duties for such managers, because the business of this type of health care is changing with such rapidity and regularity. Elements that are particularly important when developing this business acumen include research, product development, pricing, utilization review, and contracting.

Research

Research entails a continuous effort to determine the needs and desires of payers and is essential to a market-driven product. The key questions to be considered are: What do payers want and need, and are those wants and needs being adequately met? What is the competition for provision of those services? What are the costs (not prices) of the desired services at the hospital? What are the hospital's information storage and reporting capabilities?

Product Development

The products that research shows to be necessary, deliverable, and cost-effective should include types of programs and services, information needs, patient conveniences, and reporting mechanisms (including the rapidly growing field of outpatient UR). Products range from drug screenings and employee physicals to sports medicine and occupational care to wellness and employee assistance programs. Many of these are conducive to joint ventures with physicians, community agencies (for example, the local YMCA), employers, and even competitors. Services can include fast-track admission procedures as well as training care givers in patient relations. Information needs usually entail the ability to provide any financial and statistical data regarding the patients served in any variety of cross-variant formats. Patient conveniences include (in addition to rapid admission and guest relations) a minimum amount of paperwork. Reporting mechanisms are a function of the information capabilities, but also include systems that will, for example, guarantee rapid "first report of injury" information to employee supervisors.

Pricing

There are cases in which a hospital may decide to use a service as a "loss leader" or "feeder" that does not need to generate revenue. This is an increasingly risky venture, as shrinking hospital operating margins are taking away the ability to subsidize such programs. In the great majority of cases, the ambulatory care program will be expected to at least meet costs, if not generate a reasonable profit. This means that costs must be known and monitored carefully. Hospitals have not been known for effective cost accounting techniques, largely because the only cost accounting that many hospitals were forced to do in the past was for Medicare, which paid on a cost-plus basis and had its own systems for determining costs. Knowledge of all costs (direct and indirect, fixed and variable) allows a baseline to be drawn for purposes of pricing. Assuming that costs must be met, prices must be higher than costs. This sounds very basic, and it is, but hospitals frequently have been guilty of inadequate cost accounting, which can rapidly lead to financial disaster.

Other issues that are encountered frequently in pricing health care services are standards of quality and competitiveness. Not only must costs be met, but the resultant prices must be competitive if any volume is to be realized. Presumably, a standard of quality has been determined to be necessary for the service, and that standard in turn translates to costs and therefore to price. Quality is certainly a strong consideration for payers when purchasing health care, but within reason. If prices that both cover costs and are competitive cannot be developed, a number of questions need to be asked:

1. Are the costs a result of a level of quality that cannot be compromised without affecting patient care? In other words, is the proposed service a "Cadillac" version when the payer only needs and wants a simpler service? This is a common dilemma in health care, when well-meaning clinicians insist that esoteric services are essential components of a product. The hospital may then be faced with a situation in which a high-quality product has no consumers, which helps no one.
2. If it is determined that the elements of a level of quality cannot be compromised, are those elements quantifiable, explainable to a lay person, and of sufficient merit to justify (to the payer) a price that meets costs but is not competitive?
3. If the answer to the second question is no, does the hospital really want to offer a service that either will lose money or have no volume?

Utilization Review

Although mentioned briefly as an element of a salable product, outpatient utilization review deserves special mention because it is the real means by which cost savings will be realized by the payer. Discounts will result in only temporary savings to a payer, because increases in costs to the provider ultimately will be passed on to the consumer. The reduction of demand (accomplished through employee assistance programs and wellness programs), and the careful review of the resources used for those needing health care (UR) are the "only medicines that treat the disease, rather than the symptoms." Preventive measures are self-explanatory, but outpatient UR is a relatively new and growing field.

Outpatient UR is hard to perform because of the volume of patients and the difficulty in gathering and retrieving the necessary data. Emergency care, for example, does not lend itself to preadmission screening or concurrent review of care. Additionally, there is little consensus on criteria or methods for outpatient UR. In the case of ambulatory ("same-day") surgery, some of the screening criteria and second opinions that have been developed for inpatient surgeries can be used. Industrial/occupational health programs can use "case management" services in the same way in which concurrent review is utilized for inpatients. Other than those examples, though, there is little that is standardized.

The task of the ambulatory care manager, then, is to develop criteria that can work for the individual ambulatory care program to ensure appropriate use, and then develop systems that will allow those criteria to be used. For example, the outpatient physical therapy department might notice that virtually all cases of certain types of back injuries respond well to a certain course of treatment within a certain period of time. The criteria might be that such injuries require justification for any other type of treatment, and that cases that are not responsive within the normal time period must be reviewed by the physician rather than allowed to proceed endlessly. The system would then require notification of the physicians who were not already aware of the requirements of treatment modality and time limits. The system would assume that physicians who refer patients frequently to physical therapy would have been involved in the development of the criteria.

Contracting

Once a product has been developed and implemented and its support systems (billing, UR, marketing) have been defined, the relationship with payers can be cultivated to increase market share. The marketing department (if one exists) may have a plan for the general public or local businesses. The ambulatory care manager must still work closely with marketing, though, to answer questions raised by employers and third-party payers. Many hospitals now have ADS contracting departments that develop leads and answer questions regarding contracting. The ambulatory care manager should work with this department and with the finance department to provide information on costs and volume capacities and to answer technical questions for payers. The ambulatory care staff must also be aware, of course, of existing contracts and their terms.

In the absence of a marketing or contracting department, managed care agreements are generally handled by the finance department, which tends to concentrate on the inpatient side. If this is the case, the ambulatory care manager should exercise more initiative to increase volume through contracts. This involves a number of steps:

1. Develop a case for ambulatory care programs. Identify the strengths and desirable aspects, particularly in comparison to competitors. This would include prices, any fast-track systems, UR capabilities, location, reporting mechanisms, references, and types of services.
2. Work with finance to know as many of the true costs (fully allocated to include overhead) as possible. Develop a plan for contracting—how much of a discount can the hospital afford to give? What volume should be assured for each level of discount?

How much risk is the hospital willing to take; that is, which "global" (per-case or per-procedure) rates can be negotiated? Which services have little competition and therefore should not be discounted? What is a reasonable contract term?

3. Determine who will be responsible for negotiation and for "portfolio management" (keeping track of the contracts; renegotiating at the appropriate time; disseminating contract terms to billing, admission, and other affected departments; and so forth). If the ambulatory care manager is given that responsibility, steps 4 through 9 are also necessary.

4. With the assistance of finance or marketing, develop a list of union locals and self-insured companies in the area that represent sufficient potential patient volume to warrant a contractual arrangement. From that list, identify those that do not currently contract for ambulatory care through hospitalwide contracts. Typically, a hospitalwide contract would include emergency services, although outpatient diagnostic centers often are not stipulated, even if they are covered services under the payer's plan. If there is competition for those services, it may be of value to contact those payers that have been identified as meeting these criteria. The contact person will usually be the personnel director or benefits coordinator. "Those services" mean services that may not be included in a hospital's contract and those that could be contracted outside the hospital contract. "These criteria" refer to payers who: (a) have excluded certain services (or not included them) in a hospital's contract; but (b) are willing to contract "on the side" with the manager for the previously excluded service.

5. Before making contact, review the decisions made with finance regarding discount limits and related matters so that general terms can be discussed at the time of the meeting, in which the case and the proposed arrangement are presented. Also review with legal counsel any particular concerns that should be addressed. This would include termination clauses, access to records, verification of eligibility, and other points that might come up in the negotiating process. (The legal department can later handle the nonservice elements, such as liability insurance, hold-harmless clauses, litigation venue, and so forth. It may be possible to develop a generic agreement that can serve as a model and basis for negotiation.)

6. The process of negotiation is complex and can require experience, training, and skills not discussed in this chapter, but a discussion of the services, needs, and characteristics of each party is usually a good place to start. The information gathered during the initial session can be used later to fine-tune the arrangement. It will be rare that an agreement can be reached in one session.

7. For review of information gathered during the initial contact with the local payer, a checklist or "screen" of potential contract provisions is of value (figure 8-5). This same screen can also be used to evaluate requests for participation from insurance companies and PPO/HMO brokers. (Generally, it is not strategically wise to solicit business from insurance companies or brokers; it reduces the leverage of the provider in receiving information and in negotiating fees.)

8. The agreement reached must be disseminated to those departments and personnel that will need to be aware of the terms—especially admitting, billing, UR, finance, and administration. Development of a distribution list, a standard format for the terms, and a contracts portfolio list or file also is necessary to administrate these agreements effectively.

9. Each account needs to be monitored periodically to ensure that services are provided, reports are complete and timely, and problems are resolved. This can be done by the ambulatory care manager or by the marketing account executive, if such a position exists within the organization. The information gathered from this monitoring ensures adequate evaluation of service capabilities and a strong basis for renegotiation at the end of the contract term.

Conclusion

Health care reimbursement by managed care plans is a dynamic and rapidly emerging industry that is changing the ways in which health care is delivered in the United States. This trend shows no sign of slowing, much less reversing, regardless of whether or not mandatory employer-paid insurance or some form of nationalized health care is implemented in the foreseeable future. The changes in health care delivery will be most noticeable in the area of ambulatory care, and this will continue to provide the challenge to ambulatory care managers to remain innovative and knowledgeable in order to survive and lead in health care.

References

1. Etheredge, M. L. S. *Collaborative Care: Nursing Case Management.* Chicago: American Hospital Publishing, 1989, p. 3.

2. Easterbrook, G. The revolution in medicine. *Newsweek,* Jan. 26, 1987, pp. 40–74.

3. Letsch, S. W., Levit, K. R., and Waldo, D. R. National health expenditures, 1987. *Health Care Financing Review* 10(2), Winter 1988.

Figure 8-5. PPO/HMO Contract Screen—General—Memorial Hospitals Association/MediPLUS Health Plans, Inc.

Contract name: _____

Date reviewed: _____ Reviewed by: _____

Payer/Broker

1. Financial conditions
2. Organization/control
3. Track record, provider client references
4. Management
5. Service area
6. Target demographics and existing population
7. Types of groups (insurers, employees/trust funds)
8. Other contracts with MHA/MediPLUS?
9. Marketing plan

Plan

1. Preexisting conditions allowed?
2. Incentives (differential not less than 20%)
3. Payer, TPA

Contract

1. UR plan and policy retroactive denial? Cost?
2. Cash flow (days—10/30)
3. Periodic interim payment (PIP)
4. Term/termination
5. Definitions of terms
6. Rates, stop-loss administrative fee?
7. Exclusivity, preferred/nonpreferred rates?
8. Inclusion/exclusion of physician fees, durable take-home goods, implantables, prostheses, TPA, cardiac catheterization, MRI, lithotripsy, ambulance
9. Services included, inventory
10. Litigation venue
11. Late payment provision
12. Contract date, window
13. Indemnification/hold harmless
14. Third-party beneficiaries
15. Access to records
16. Other

Source: Memorial Hospitals Association, Inc., 1989.

Glossary of Common Insurance and Managed Care Terms

Competitive Medical Plan (CMP) — Operates under the same criteria as an HMO, except that it does not require federal qualification; can offer variable benefit programs and can "experience rate" its products.

Health Maintenance Organization (HMO) — An organization licensed by the state; is federally qualified, offering a specific range of hospital, physician, laboratory, and X-ray services; is at financial risk and is compensated by its members at a predetermined rate.

Indemnity (FFS) — Traditional fully insured billed-charge and fee-for-service medical coverage. Providers bill at usual and customary rates and are reimbursed for a percentage of their fees for each service performed.

Insured Product Option (IPO) — A joint venture of insurance companies and provider networks to offer a variety of options (PPO, CMP, HMO, managed programs) to employers. The joint venture of VHA and Aetna to develop Partners National Health Plans is an example of an IPO.

Managed FFS — Indemnity programs that attempt to control costs through utilization review (second surgical opinions, preadmission screening, and so forth).

Managed Premium Product/Reserve Capacity — Also known as M3POs. A variation of PPO coverage that includes assumption of financial risk from the provider network and a guarantee of premium rates to the purchaser in excess of one year. Providers accept risk in the form of amounts withheld from the rates pending success of the plan in meeting its financial goals.

Medicare Capitation — Individual coverage offered through HMOs and CMPs at low or zero monthly premiums.

Medicare Supplement — Individual coverage designed to cover dollar amounts not paid by Medicare. Also known as "Medigap" insurance.

Preferred Provider Organization (PPO) — A network of hospitals and physicians who have individually contracted with purchasers to accept set reimbursement rates in exchange for higher patient volume.

Third-Party Administrator (TPA) — A service designed to offer bundled or unbundled administrative services, including billing, claims processing (health, drug, dental, vision), utilization review, and data analysis to self-insured customers.

Source: Memorial Hospitals Association, Inc., 1989.

Chapter 9

The Future of Ambulatory Care

Diane M. Howard

The ambulatory care industry has been described as a $45 billion industry with an excess of 300 million visits annually.[1] The breadth of ambulatory care services ranges from hospital outpatient clinics, emergency services, and group practice—long the traditional delivery routes—to freestanding ambulatory care facilities, ambulatory surgery, home care, hospices, managed care activities, and a host of diagnostic and therapeutic services.

At last report, there are over 4,242 hospitals that offer ambulatory care services, over 2,400 Medicare-certified home health agencies, over 1,000 ambulatory surgery centers, 9,000 physician office laboratories performing over 400,000 tests annually, over 3,300 freestanding ambulatory care centers, over 1,900 hospice programs, over 88,300 physicians practicing in a group setting, and over 650 operational HMOs enrolling a total of over 30 million people.[2]

Ambulatory care has grown so quickly since the introduction of the prospective payment system (PPS) in 1983 that the nature of the services being offered are difficult to quantify. The system is so fragmented and diverse and has so many competing interests that it is almost impossible to control. Control of expenditures and utilization, however, is precisely what is in store for ambulatory care.

The introduction of the prospective payment system with the Tax Equity and Fiscal Responsibility Act of 1983 reduced Medicare expenditures associated with hospitalization. Although inpatient occupancy was reduced from 75 percent to 64 percent from 1980 to 1988 and average length of stay was reduced from 7.6 to 7.1 days over the same period, Medicare Part B, which pays for outpatient services, increased by 18 percent.[3] In addition, the annual growth rate in inpatient revenues from 1973 to 1988 was 6.1 percent, whereas outpatient revenues increased 16.9 percent in the same period.[4]

The mushrooming of ambulatory care expenditures and the need to control them will necessitate the restructuring of ambulatory care.

Whereas the decade of the 1980s introduced significant health care change, the prospect for the 1990s is unclear. Hospitals have expanded their ambulatory care programming to compensate for their inpatient revenue losses due to PPS and to respond to the insurance industry's search for lower-cost alternatives to inpatient care. Hospital diversification into ambulatory care or the repackaging of out-of-hospital services to achieve financial goals had mixed reviews, depending upon the geographic area, the resources devoted to the initiatives, physician support, and client acceptance of the enterprise.

In a 1988 survey conducted by an American Hospital Association magazine, *Hospitals,* data indicate that seven diversification strategies produced a profit—freestanding outpatient diagnostic centers, inpatient rehabilitation centers, outpatient psychiatric centers, women's medicine programs, industrial medical clinics, and substance abuse treatment centers.[5] Although diversification prospects have been promising, the long-term growth of ambulatory care can no longer be separated from broader health care issues.

Issues Affecting the Future of Ambulatory Care

Issues of homelessness, substance abuse, acquired immunodeficiency syndrome (AIDS), and a growing senior citizen population will change the face of health care and will have a dramatic effect on the future of hospital-based ambulatory care—the key access point to the hospital. In the 1980s there was a concentration of resources on profitable entrepreneurial initiatives in ambulatory care, but in the 1990s, initiatives will be devoted to developing more ambulatory care alternatives to inpatient rehabilitation and long-term care. Prognostication for the future of ambulatory care, as with anything else, is merely speculative, but attention should be directed to the following:

- The United States, like most industrial and developing countries, is struggling to regulate health care. The health care industry during the Reagan years (1980–1988) was marked by entrepreneurism, a free-market philosophy, and cost reduction. The health care legacy of the Bush presidency is unknown as yet, but it is clear that health care will be more of a priority for President Bush than it was for the Reagan administration. Upon entering office, Bush indicated that one of his priorities will be to improve the efficiency, effectiveness, and quality of the U.S. health care system.
- The emphasis on budget deficit reduction by an estimated $127 billion for fiscal year 1990 will have a significant impact on the expansion and

control of health care spending.[6] President Bush's budget projects Medicare spending will be reduced by $5 billion, with $3.3 billion of that coming from hospitals.[7]

- State initiatives in health care are under way in the absence of a federal commitment to health care spending. Where federal health care gaps exist, states will play a greater health care role. New York's Governor Mario Cuomo, acknowledging a $2 billion state deficit, committed state resources to fight drugs and increase basic welfare grants.[8] As an example, New York is setting up two small pilot programs to allow some low-income families and small businesses to buy subsidized health insurance.[9] The state of Washington will pay up to 90 percent of the cost of health insurance for selected families whose incomes are less than double the poverty level. About 30,000 Washingtonians, 4 percent of those who have no health insurance, will be covered in the first five years, and state officials say they hope to expand the plan if it proves successful. Massachusetts law requires employers to participate in a health insurance pool. The program is taking effect in phases, and it currently covers 7,600 people. Pennsylvania, California, and Hawaii are also experimenting with state health care initiatives. An article in the *New York Times* indicated that health care for lower-middle-class citizens has become a nonpartisan issue, much as unemployment was in the 1930s.[10]
- There will be other state initiatives to resolve pressing health care issues. New York State issued rules that require hospitals to move patients out of emergency rooms quickly by either transferring them to inpatient beds, discharging them, or ensuring that they receive the kind of care they would receive in a hospital inpatient ward.[11]

A host of health care and social problems are threatening to pierce the integrity of our social welfare and health care safety net. These include homelessness, drug and alcohol abuse, AIDS, an aging population, and ethnic shifts in population. Each of these phenomena will place a unique demand upon the structural components of the health delivery system, especially in the ambulatory care arena. Health care providers must find creative ways to accommodate the needs of these populations so as to lessen the financial and organizational burdens they will impose on the health care system. The following statistics illustrate the issues raised by the aforementioned health care and social problems:

- The problem of the homeless will not simply go away; it will continue to be a growing national phenomenon. A variety of estimates indicate that there are 350,000 to 4 million homeless Americans.[12] An estimated 25 percent to 50 percent of these are mentally ill and are homeless because of the nationwide push for deinstitutionalization.

- The National Institute on Drug Abuse (NIDA) and the National Institute on Alcohol Abuse and Alcoholism (NIAAA) estimate that at least 10 percent of the work force is affected by alcoholism or drug addiction. An additional 10 percent to 15 percent is affected by substance abuse by an immediate family member.[13]
- A recent estimate by the Alcohol, Drug Abuse, and Mental Health Administration indicates that alcohol and drug abuse together cost the country more than $140 billion annually, including $100 billion in lost productivity.[14]
- Alcoholism is a disease that affects a large portion of the population; it is estimated that 10 million Americans experience some problems resulting from their drinking habits.[15]
- Twenty years ago, there were about 10,000 cocaine users in the United States; ten years ago, there were 100,000. Current estimates range from 5 million to over 20 million cocaine users, resulting in fivefold increases in the number of cocaine-related emergency room vists, admissions to drug treatment programs, and deaths.[16]
- The National Institute on Drug Abuse estimated that in 1986, 3 million people abused cocaine regularly, more than five times the number addicted to heroin.[17]
- The 1990 fiscal year budget formally submitted by President Bush proposed a $424.4 billion allocation for health and human services that includes a 30 percent increase in spending on AIDS. The administration recommended spending $2.5 billion on AIDS, including $1.6 billion for research, education, and prevention, and $925 million for treatment and other assistance for AIDS victims.[18]
- It is estimated that there are presently between 1 million and 1.5 million people in the United States who have been infected with the AIDS virus. Estimates provided by the Centers for Disease Control (CDC) project that by 1991 at least 340,000 people in this country will have been diagnosed with AIDS and that 109,000 of these persons will be alive at that time. It is also anticipated that in 1991 at least 1 percent of all hospital beds in the nation will be occupied by AIDS patients and that treatment costs for AIDS will consume more than 3 percent of the national health care budget.[19]
- There were 66,464 cases of AIDS reported to the CDC between June 1, 1981, and July 4, 1988. Of these, 69.9 percent were homosexual or bisexual men, 20.8 percent were heterosexual men, 7.8 percent were women, and 1.6 percent were children under 13 years of age.[20]
- People aged 55 and older represent over one-fifth of the U.S. population and more than one-third of all householders. This large market consists of four segments: the older population (aged 55 to 64), the elderly (65 to 74), the aged (75 to 84), and the very old (85 and older). Whereas the total U.S. population is projected to grow 19 percent

between 1987 and 2015, the mature population will grow fully 62 percent.[21]

The U.S. health care system is not prepared to deal with this elderly population or the broader nature of the services they will need. Ambulatory care services will need to be expanded to allow access to adult day-care services, respite care, and ambulatory rehabilitation services that will require integration with home care and long-term care services.

Because of the fragmentation in the current health care system, independent programmatic service units have developed in hospitals to cater to narrow market niches. This fascination with narrow markets will have to be discontinued as the need grows for a more rational and integrated system to serve the growing population of elderly persons.

- Ethnic shifts in the population will also have an impact on the structure and delivery of health care services. The growth in the Hispanic population, especially the influx of non-English-speaking Hispanics into urban areas, will necessitate the use of bilingual personnel in service areas typically accessed by newly arrived Hispanics—emergency rooms, outpatient clinics, and neighborhood health centers. Since 1980, the Hispanic population has increased by 34 percent, in comparison to an increase of only 7 percent for the non-Hispanic population. The Hispanic population is projected to increase by 34 percent between 1988 and 2000, the white population by 7 percent, and the black population by 16 percent.[22]

Predictions for the Future of Ambulatory Care

Because of the diversity of ambulatory care programs, an assessment of how these and other issues will affect particular programs is useful. What follows is an assessment of how the issues and trends will affect emergency services, hospital-based ambulatory care programs, and ambulatory care diversification ventures.

Emergency Services

The emergency department, long considered the access point to the hospital on an unscheduled basis, will continue to be just that for the foreseeable future. Currently, there are 5,272 hospitals providing emergency medical services; 1,042 of these are in the trauma system.[23]

Teenage pregnancies and infant illness, AIDS and other sexually transmitted diseases, chronic illnesses among the aged, and chemical dependency are just a few of the causes of mortality and morbidity being seen in the

U.S. health care delivery system.[24] When the increasing numbers of home-less people and the 37 million uninsured and underinsured are factored in, it is clear that the health care delivery system will be forced to explore new ways of structuring to accommodate the divergent clinical, social, and psychological needs of these populations. The hospital emergency department will continue to be the clinical manager of unscheduled patient visits and will seek ways to reduce its exposure to nonpaying patients.

Hospitals will have to look closely at the indigent caseload entering through their emergency departments and pursue one of the following courses:

1. Hospitals will reduce their exposure to uninsured and underinsured patients by eliminating emergency services.
2. If emergency services are maintained, hospitals will establish link-ages, where appropriate, with other hospitals in order to share a proportion of the indigent caseload.
3. Hospitals will add or strengthen case management expertise in the emergency departments by the use of social workers, who can iden-tify community services for assistive living, thus taking the nonclin-ical burden from nursing and medical staffs. Assistive living includes housing, food, and primary care providers that are not emergency-department-based, and identification of self-help programs that allow the client to pursue health care alternatives independent from the hospital.
4. Hospitals will develop the emergency department as an integrated care provider with other hospital-based ambulatory care programs. Those patient conditions that are nonemergency will be directed to hospital-based programs where the intensity of services is less, as is the cost.
5. Hospitals will reverse their commitment, if a commitment was made, to participate in a trauma system. Depending upon patient mix, loca-tion, and commitment to community services, some hospitals may find it economically unattractive to treat the many underinsured and uninsured patients who traditionally present through a trauma sys-tem. Declining to participate in a trauma system will reduce this vital service to the community. Prominent examples of this trend are hospi-tals in metropolitan areas in the states of California, Florida, and Illinois.
6. If many hospitals opt out of providing emergency department ser-vices, those hospitals that retain their emergency service will see their patient volume increase. Physicians practicing in these hospi-tal emergency departments will require increased liability coverage, the cost of which will be passed on to the patient or absorbed by the hospital.

7. Hospitals will see patient satisfaction decline and delays increase as emergency departments are deluged with various nonurgent and urgent conditions.

8. Those hospitals that experience increased AIDS and substance abuse cases will see a higher degree of staff burnout than they have encountered in the past and higher-than-usual staff vacancies.

9. To decrease the emergency department occupancy rate of the homeless and their subsequent rate of hospital admissions, state and local home health services will be made available, along with the appropriate social services. These will be state and local initiatives, but will not be national in scope because of the budget deficit.

10. Rural hospitals will find it difficult to maintain enough of an operating margin to stay in the acute care business and will consider converting hospitals to ambulatory care facilities with emergency services capabilities. Rural hospitals will establish referral mechanisms to larger acute care facilities and will find it even more difficult to recruit physicians and nurses in this new hospital role.

11. Emergency departments will continue to compete with the urgent care market. However, the latter will fall on hard times because for many the primary care market has proved to be too insubstantial for long-term growth needs. Hospital emergency departments that have fast-tracking, an attractive physical plant, fast turnaround from laboratory and radiology services, a competent clinical staff, and patient education and quality assurance programs will continue to meet the competition from nonhospital providers.

Hospital-Based Ambulatory Care Programs

Hospital-based ambulatory care programs have evolved over the years. Traditionally, the programs were financially subsidized by hospitals and emphasized physician training. The role of hospital-based ambulatory care programs, originally designated as clinics, has expanded to provide training for other clinical disciplines as well. The expansion of these programs was accelerated by the introduction of Medicare and Medicaid in the late 1960s and no further significant changes occurred until the introduction of the Medicare prospective payment system in 1983. In most cases prior to 1983, hospital-based ambulatory care operated with no financial incentives for the hospital or medical staff; the programs provided access to the hospital and fulfilled a teaching function. Medicare PPS changed hospital-based programs by encouraging hospitals to reorganize their ambulatory programs.

After 1983, the focus of hospital-based ambulatory care changed. No longer was it enough for these programs to simply provide a site for educational training; the programs also were expected to increase revenues, provide hospital visibility in the community, increase market share, and increase inpatient occupancy.[25] As entrepreneurism invaded the hospital, more ambulatory care programs were organized away from hospitals and away from hospital overhead allocation and management bureaucracy. However, as these programs proliferated under hospital ownership, so did the friction between the hospital and its medical staff.

The programs that generated marginal revenues because of an attractive insurance climate for ambulatory care catered to a private patient population that was spun out of the hospital. Freestanding outpatient diagnostic centers, freestanding outpatient surgery, and programs in industrial medicine, women's medicine, psychiatric care, home health care, substance abuse, and cardiac rehabilitation became the new wave of ambulatory care programs and were designated as diversification ventures.[26]

Along with emergency departments, hospital-based ambulatory care programs struggled to compete with the more prosperous programs located off the hospital campus. The future viability of hospital-based ambulatory care programs will rest with the advent of a proposed 1991 prospective payment system for ambulatory care.

A January 1989 survey was conducted by the American Hospital Association's Society for Ambulatory Care Professionals to ascertain the current impact of ambulatory surgery payment changes and to identify potential management concerns about the conversion of ambulatory care programs to a prospective payment system by 1991. The survey identified the following statistics:

1. The approximate number of man-hours required to convert a facility to the Current Procedural Terminology (CPT-4) billing system is 229.
2. The average number of full-time equivalents (FTEs) added to the admitting and billing function is 1.4, with an average annual salary of $11,585.
3. The average number of FTEs added to the medical records function is 1.59, with an average annual salary of $20,165.
4. On average, respondents indicated that 1.7 FTEs would be necessary on a permanent basis to accomplish this CPT-4 coding requirement, and that 1.0 FTE would be reassigned from another hospital unit to accomplish the CPT-4 coding function.
5. The Medicare outpatient payment system has added an average of four days to the hospital accounts receivables; 60 percent of the respondents thought that this delay would be permanent.

Fully 60 percent of the reporting hospitals indicated that they had made operational changes to accommodate the changes in ambulatory surgery payment. The operational changes in rank order by strategy included group purchasing, purchasing of less costly supplies, employee input into planning, flexible staff scheduling, employee cross-training, increased use of part-time workers, and standardized supply ordering.

In addition, 60 percent of the respondents indicated that they would not undertake certain operational changes, including, in rank order, salary reductions, employee benefit reductions, job reclassification, union decertification, reduction of a commitment to uncompensated care, incentive programs for nonmedical staff, staff reductions, incentive programs for physicians, and linkage of pay to productivity. The majority commented that more time was needed to assess the full impact of payment changes. When a thorough assessment is made, however, one suspects that a reduction in human resources and protecting the hospital's exposure to high-risk nonpaying patients will be strategies selected by some hospitals.

The survey revealed that in 1988, 56 percent of respondents added ambulatory care services and 44 percent eliminated some services. In planning for the future, 55 percent indicated they would add services, whereas 45 percent planned to eliminate services. During 1988 and 1989, the services that hospitals added and planned to add included diagnostic imaging, hospice, emergency or urgent care, general radiology, occupational therapy, and home health. Although respondents indicated that dental services was the only program that had been eliminated from their programs, the list of eliminated programs is expected to grow as hospitals assess their financial position in hospital-based ambulatory care programming. Additional services being considered for ambulatory care expansion are diet centers, mobile laser services, emergency medical services, geriatric services, oncology programming, and pain clinics.

The future of hospital-based programming will require a reduction in hospital overhead, 40 percent of survey respondents indicated that they would place greater emphasis on freestanding facilities, with 88 percent emphasizing shared department activities, and 87 percent emphasizing more efficient energy use.

Because the ambulatory PPS system is still being developed, the future of hospital-based ambulatory care programming is unclear. If inpatient prospective payment is any indication of what will happen to outpatient services, the following prognostications can be made:

1. Hospital-based ambulatory care programming will be driven to provide a teaching environment for medical residents in internal medicine and pediatrics by the Bureau of Health Professions, which requires that 25 percent of resident training occur in a "continuity setting" or a primary care setting.
2. This graduate medical education initiative will make hospital-based ambulatory care programs less attractive to private paying patients, who want care from an attending physician in a relatively short time span.

3. Hospital management will struggle to make these programs financially viable and will consider introducing productivity standards and providing incentives for efficiency.

4. Much like emergency departments, hospital-based ambulatory care programs will limit their exposure to indigent patients and will exist as teaching and training environments for physicians, nurses, and allied health professionals. Medical social workers and case managers will direct patients with chronic conditions to community resources for monitoring.

5. Hospital-based ambulatory care programs will be absorbed into physician group practices affiliated with hospitals. Where privatizing the ambulatory care programs is not possible, small ambulatory care enterprises will exist. Community utilization and hospital commitment to the enterprise will be primary reasons to continue the services.

Ambulatory Care Diversification Ventures

Dean Coddington, a well-known health care strategist, defines diversification as a strategy that attempts to spread financial risk by taking advantage of new market opportunities.[27] In the context of ambulatory care, diversification is an activity that allows the hospital to increase gross revenue, increase market share, increase inpatient occupancy, meet the challenge of competition, respond to demographic changes, and provide a community service. The activity is usually away from the hospital campus and has a financial and administrative management structure that is independent of the hospital. *Hospitals* magazine ranked the success of services in the following order:[28]

- Freestanding outpatient diagnostic services
- Freestanding outpatient surgery
- Industrial medicine

Several prognostications for the future follow:

1. Ambulatory care programs will continue to maintain the interest of hospitals for the foreseeable future because of their profitability.

2. Certain programs will be introduced, but others will be eliminated after failing to produce an anticipated benefit or financial effect. The life cycle for each venture will be variable.

3. As the prospective payment system is developed, units of ambulatory care service will be rebundled along a continuum to integrate patient care and to meet the standards specified by the new ambulatory care payment system.

4. Hospital management of diversification ventures will be strengthened as hospital medical staffs reduce their resistance to these ventures.
5. Diversification ventures that are not patient-care oriented will have their nonprofit status revoked and will find it difficult to compete with for-profit enterprises.

Future Issues for Consideration

The U.S. health care system is at war with itself. There are so many competing interests — hospitals, managed care organizations, physicians, nurses, allied health professionals, third-party payers — that no one entity is capable of organizing the system so that resources are equitably distributed and access to the system is preserved. The one real hope is that health care will become more of a priority at the national level and that the federal government, through its financing mechanism, will slowly encourage the restructuring of the system, much as it did with the introduction of Medicare, Medicaid, the Health Maintenance Organization (HMO) Act, and prospective payment. What will be needed, however, is a rational approach that integrates the philosophies of the past into a broader and more equitable system that preserves the private practice of medicine.

References

1. American Hospital Association. *Trends in Medicare Expenditures.* Office of Health Finance and Data Analysis, Apr. 21, 1989, attachment 1. Chicago: AHA, 1989.

2. Hospital Data Center. Interview. American Hospital Association, May 1989, and Ambulatory care growth continues. *Outreach* 10(1):1, Jan.–Feb. 1989.

3. Howard, D. M. *Past Experiences and Future Directions in Ambulatory Care.* Chicago: AHA, 1988, p. 17.

4. National Hospital Panel Survey, Office of Health Finance and Data Analysis, Mar. 1989. Chicago: American Hospital Association.

5. Sabatino, F. G. The diversification success story continues: survey. *Hospitals* 63(1):27, Jan. 5, 1989.

6. Talks by Darman show Bush's plans to handle budget. *New York Times,* Jan. 5, 1989, p. 1.

7. Editorials. *Modern Healthcare,* Feb. 24, 1989.

8. Mr. Cuomo's priorities, and their price. *New York Times,* Jan. 5, 1989, p. 20.

9. Egan, T. A state offers working poor insurance aid. *New York Times,* Jan. 2, 1989, p. 1.

10. Egan, p. 1.

11. French, H. New York hospitals fear problems with new rules. *New York Times,* Jan. 4, 1989, p. 10.

12. Wagner, L. Offering care to the poorest of the poor. *Modern Healthcare,* Dec. 23, 1988, p. 24.

13. Wrich, J. T. Beyond testing: coping with drugs at work. *EAP Digest* 9(1):56, Nov.-Dec. 1988.

14. Wrich, p. 57.

15. Sullivan-Chin, M., and Chin, J. C. Reaching unseen victims: adult children of alcoholics. *EAP Digest* 8(4):51-2, 63, May/June 1988.

16. Larson, J. W. LifePLUS transitional recovery unit. *EAP Digest* 8(4):28, 70-1, May/June 1988.

17. Gawin, F. H., and Ellinwood, E. H., Jr. Cocaine and other stimulants: actions, abuse and treatment. *New England Journal of Medicine* 318(18):1173-82, May 5, 1988.

18. Personal communication. American Hospital Association, Washington Office, May 1989.

19. Dunham, N. C. *Task Force on HIV/AIDS and Health Service Administration Education.* Rockville, MD: Department of Health and Human Services, Bureau of Health Professions, 1988.

20. Selik, R. M., Castro, K. G., and Pappaioanou, M. Distribution of AIDS cases by racial/ethnic group and exposure category, June 1, 1981-July 4, 1988. *Morbidity and Mortality Weekly Report* 37, suppl. no. SS-3, 1988.

21. Lazer, W., and Shaw, E. H. How older Americans spend their money. *American Demographics* 9(8):36-41, Sept. 1987.

22. U.S. Bureau of the Census. Current Population Reports, Series P-25, No. 1018. *Projections of the Population of the United States by Age, Sex, and Race; 1988-2080.* Washington, DC: U.S. Bureau of the Census, 1989.

23. Ambulatory care growth continues. *Outreach* 10(1):1, Jan.-Feb. 1989.

24. Zimmerman, E. Environmental assessment for society for ambulatory care professionals. Unpublished research, 1988.

25. Howard, D. M. *New Business Development in Ambulatory Care: Exploring Diversification Options.* Chicago: American Hospital Publishing, 1988, p. 17.

26. Sabatino, p. 27.

27. Howard, D. M. *New Business Development in Ambulatory Care,* p. 4.

28. Sabatino, p. 27.

Part Two

Innovative Ambulatory Care Programs

Chapter 10

Integrating Inpatient and Outpatient Services in One Building

William C. Mason

By 1984, the management of Baptist Medical Center (BMC) in Jacksonville, Florida, was feeling both internal and external pressure to construct additional facilities. The center's personnel recognized that there were some things that they needed to be doing better internally. They also perceived a changing external market that was moving into unfamiliar times. The management team knew that it must look into the future and meet the needs of several publics that obviously would be in existence in the next few years. It was then that the Baptist Medical Pavilion began to evolve.

Creating the Plan

The medical staff needed more space and updated facilities and equipment, especially in obstetrics (OB). The center did not necessarily need more beds; it did need more adequate facilities. Out-of-town patients needed special amenities to enhance their visits. Everyone agreed that there were half as many parking spaces as were needed. The shift in emphasis from inpatient care to outpatient care was obviously here to stay. Outpatient services were growing fast, with pressures from all sides brought about by the shift to the inpatient prospective payment system. In 1984, BMC's proportion of outpatient business was 55 percent and rising. Also, the large out-of-town caseload from south Georgia as well as north Florida made it even more necessary that BMC truly meet total patient needs. This meant having one campus that included:

- Outpatient laboratories, X rays, and surgery
- Physicians' offices close by, especially those utilizing building services

- Affordable overnight accommodations (such as could be provided by an on-campus hotel)
- A retail pharmacy where prescriptions could be filled quickly
- Commercial businesses that would enhance the concept of total patient care
- A good restaurant where patients and family members could eat
- A hospital immediately adjacent, in case of outpatient need
- A comprehensive health and fitness center

Baptist Medical Center was striving toward the concept of total patient care, which meant being as complete as possible—having independent outpatient services as well as inpatient services, should they be needed—in an attractive, comfortable, homelike setting with a personal atmosphere. The center was, in fact, in 1984 ready to open for bid seven stories of patient floors on top of the already-existing nine-story BMC Wolfson Tower. The patient floors were architecturally complete. These floors were to be designated for obstetrics, medicine, surgery, and pediatrics.

Separate from the seven-story addition, a physicians' office building and the sorely needed parking garage were also being planned. The problem was how to finance those three projects simultaneously. Additionally, in perspective, BMC's management team recognized that the center was in a changing market in which reimbursement patterns were not settled and in which the delivery modality was changing from inpatient to outpatient. The management team was unsure of what prospective payment would bring and did not know to what extent the delivery modalities would be changed. The pressures of alternative delivery systems had the possibility of significantly reducing BMC's patient volumes.

Furthermore, BMC was operating under several constraints; namely, the concern of adding too much debt (debt capacity), trying to accurately estimate the projected profitability of operations (which has a direct impact on debt capacity), and geographic restrictions. The center's geographic restrictions were such that, being located on a 15½-plus acre peninsula, every square foot of space was being utilized, and already there was more acreage under roof and carpark than there was in land area. It was with all these constraints that BMC was trying to respond to perceived and foreseeable needs.

Rethinking the Plan

As the magnitude of internal and external needs and pressures as well as financial and logistical constraints began to sink in, BMC's management team recognized that it might do better to rethink the whole plan. The decision-making process was arduous, and it relied a great deal on consultants who specialized in hospital medical office buildings. Finally, rather than add 7 stories to the Wolfson Tower and construct a 20-story physicians' office building with parking space, the team conceived the idea of cutting 10 floors off the plans for the physicians' building, lifting it up, and relocating OB services underneath it. The plans for the OB unit, including neonatal intensive care, were modified to fit the footprint of the physicians' office building. In the process of rethinking the ways to meet needs, management envisioned a two-floor hotel between OB and the physicians' offices—which is what was done—and The Pavilion Inn was conceived.

Financing the Plan

The center's debt capacity was a very real constraint and called for some highly creative maneuvers in order to bring the dream to fruition. As it turned out, the Pavilion was financed through tax-exempt bonds, philanthropic fund-raising, and a limited partnership. Furthermore, the physicians' office space was sold as a condominium to a limited partnership composed primarily of BMC physicians shortly after construction was begun.

The complete lower floors of the Pavilion, the shell of the top 10 floors, and the parking garage (plus an addition to the award-winning cogeneration energy center) were financed with the proceeds of more than $42 million in tax-exempt, variable-rate demand notes. (Variable-rate demand notes have an interest rate that floats on a weekly basis, but over time tracks other short-term interest rates, usually at considerably less than prime.) The physician limited partnership, debt financed through another tax-exempt bond issue, purchased the yet-to-be-built shell and financed the improvements required in order to bring the office structure to full operational status.

Baptist Medical Center also conducted a $7.5 million community-employee fund-raising campaign to provide a portion of the monies for the project. In conjunction with refinancing a 1982 bond issue in 1985, BMC developed a financial strategy to lock in a maximum rate of 8.65 percent while allowing for the positive arbitrage of over $40 million on a 1984 variable-rate financing done for the Pavilion. The technique, known as "crossover refunding," used a combination of tax-exempt revenue bonds with a fixed rate of 8.65 percent, variable-rate demand notes (which generally are one to two points below prime), and the investment management of an escrow fund equal to the principal of the variable-rate debt obligation. The current cost of the financing is 5.65 percent. It cannot exceed 8.65 percent and will always be reduced by an amount equal to the difference between investment revenue and 8.65 percent.

Facilities and Amenities of the Pavilion

The management team of Baptist Medical Center worked hard to simplify complex matters and, above all, to meet the needs of its various publics. It felt that it was responding to as many of the changes in health care delivery as could be foreseen in 1984. Obstetrics was becoming more visible and more family-oriented. The center's new strategic focus included women's services. Baptist Medical Center increased the visibility and productivity of outpatient services at a time when the whole health care delivery system was moving to accommodate the outpatient. New trends included health and fitness centers and hotels based at medical center campuses. Physicians' offices within the medical center complex offered obvious advantages to the physician, patient, and medical center. All of these services were combined in one vertical structure—the Baptist Medical Pavilion. The floor plan for the Pavilion makes for a building unique in health care in its marriage of design and function. It is a rare example of physicians' offices merged with commercial lease space, outpatient services, acute inpatient hospital facilities (including obstetrics and neonatal care), and a hotel.

In order to begin to appreciate the unusual efficiency of the building, a brief description of the 283,311-square-foot floor plan is necessary (figure 10-1):

- The first floor:
  - Outpatient laboratories, which include X ray and ECG.
  - Commercial lease enterprises, including a gift shop, travel agency, florist, pharmacy, eyewear store, hotel registration desk, and 90-seat restaurant.
- The second and third floors:
  - The *Wolfson Center for Mothers and Infants,* which offers the very latest facilities and equipment and centralizes obstetrical services. Here extra care is taken in every way possible to make the birth process more rewarding for the entire family. The labor and delivery area is specially appointed. Comfortable birthing rooms offer women with uncomplicated pregnancies the chance to experience labor, delivery, bonding, and recovery in a homelike setting. A new service offers special facilities for high-risk mothers.
  - The *Neonatal Intensive Care Unit,* located immediately adjacent to the delivery area, renders special care to critically ill and convalescing newborns. A parenting room is available so that parents can spend the night and care for their baby under the supervision of a nurse.
  - The *Postpartum Unit* offers individualized predelivery and postdelivery care to new mothers and their families in specially designed and decorated comfortable surroundings.

Figure 10-1. Pavilion Baptist Medical Center, Commercial/Outpatient, First Floor

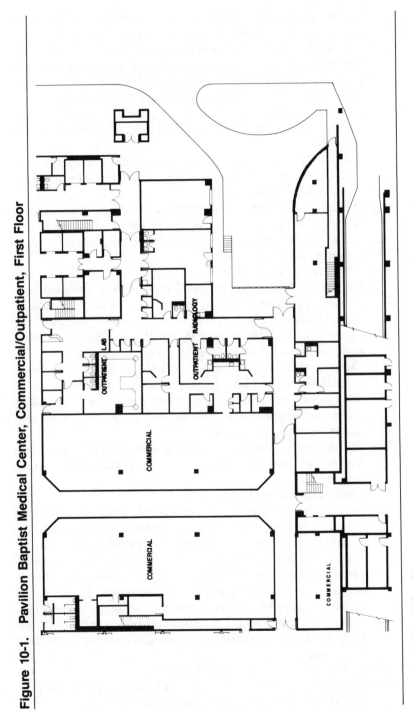

Source: Drexel Toland & Associates.

- The *Term Nursery* is a family-centered care area for newborns and their families that provides rooming-in, parenting education, and special opportunities for mother–baby nursing.
- The *Women's Resource Center* provides a library and educational programs to meet the changing life-styles of women. Nursing professionals offer a comprehensive health care program for women of all ages that emphasizes family-centered care with specialized medical and surgical technologies, including those for high-risk mothers and infants.
- The *OB/GYN Clinic* offers a full range of obstetrical services for families that cannot afford medical care from a private physician.
- The fourth floor (figure 10-2):
  - The *Ambulatory Surgical Unit* offers a comfortable setting in which healthy patients can undergo certain procedures that can be performed on the same day, thus eliminating the need for a costly overnight stay in the hospital.
- The fifth floor (figure 10-3):
  - The *Baptist Health and Fitness Center* offers a walk/jog track around the inside perimeter of the floor, a wide range of Nautilus exercise equipment, comprehensive individualized programs, and a professional staff that is degreed, experienced in exercise programming, and certified in cardiopulmonary resuscitation.
  - The *Cardiac Rehabilitation Center,* an integral part of the Southeast Heart Institute, provides professional expertise and monitoring of patients undergoing the rigorous training necessary to learn how to live a healthier and more satisfactory life after being diagnosed or treated for heart ailments.
  - The *Outpatient Physical Therapy Department* includes the sports medicine program, the back school, and outpatient orthopedic services.
- The sixth and seventh floors:
  - The *Pavilion Inn,* a 48-room hotel specially designed for patients and their families. The hotel gives patients the alternative of remaining on campus for diagnosis or treatment without incurring a costly hospital bill. It is also available for those, especially out-of-towners, who want to remain close to a hospitalized family member. The rooms are spacious, quiet, beautifully furnished, and affordable. They have climate control, telephone, and color television, and some include a refrigerator, stove, and microwave. There are special appointments for the handicapped in several of the rooms.
- The eighth through seventeenth floors:
  - The physicians' offices, which offer a beautiful view of Jacksonville as well as convenience to medical center services.

Figure 10-2. Pavilion Baptist Medical Center, Ambulatory Surgery, Fourth Floor

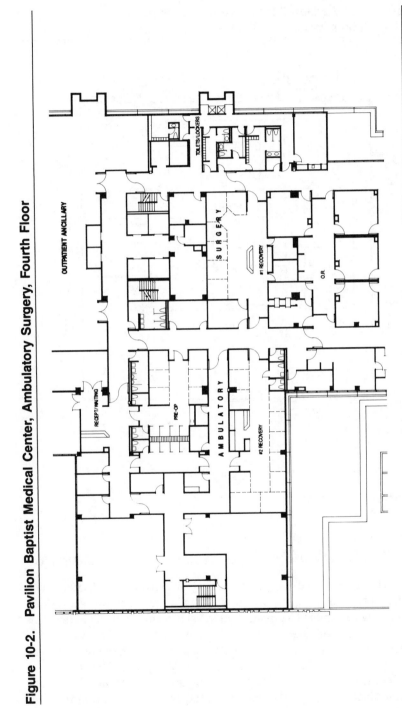

Source: Drexel Toland & Associates.

Figure 10-3. Pavilion Baptist Medical Center, Cardiac Rehabilitation and Wellness, Fifth Floor

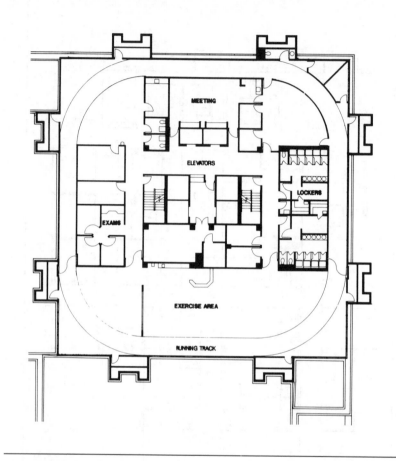

Source: Drexel Toland & Associates.

The Pavilion's First Two Years: An Assessment

The Pavilion celebrated its grand opening on September 13, 1987. The architects produced a superb design, and BMC's management was thrilled that a highly constrained, complex project such as this came out better than originally conceived. The location of the two-floor Wolfson Center for Mothers and Infants directly below obstetrician offices; the onsite outpatient laboratories; the one-floor Ambulatory Surgical Unit; the Health and Fitness Center, including the Cardiac Rehabilitation Center and Outpatient Physical Therapy (all on the same floor); the two-floor Pavilion Inn hotel;

and 10 floors of physician office space—all these combine functionally to make it an extremely efficient building.

As has been indicated, the hotel, The Pavilion Inn, serves the entire hospital community in a number of unique ways. Not only can families of patients stay in a hotel that is on the hospital campus, but also patients who come in for outpatient procedures and who do not warrant hospitalization may spend a period of recuperation next to the hospital so that if there are any complications, the patients can then be quickly admitted. The hotel also allows high-risk obstetrics patients who need to be confined to bed, and who until now were often admitted to the hospital, to spend their prenatal time, be it 2 weeks or 10, in a more "normal" environment.

One of the areas that has had a most salutary effect on BMC's operations is ambulatory surgery. With the majority of outpatient services shifting from the main hospital to the Pavilion, some pressure on staff, equipment, and, most important, patients, has been relieved. Time has been saved, especially in laboratory services. Outpatients are no longer mixed with inpatients in laboratory services, so that now there is, for all practical purposes, no waiting time. In addition, space has been created for a Day Stay unit in the main hospital where surgery or outpatient treatments can be performed. Outpatient surgery has relieved inpatient operating and recovery rooms so that personnel are able to concentrate their skills where they can be best used. Inpatient surgery is used only for the more complicated procedures. Surgery on an outpatient basis costs approximately 40 percent less than inpatient surgery. An all-inclusive fee is used so that a patient is actually quoted a price for the procedure.

Outpatient surgery can still be done in the main operating room. As a matter of fact, one of the very real advantages of the Pavilion is that the surgery department is more flexible for physicians. In the Pavilion, a physician can be offered a choice of operating rooms, so that a particular physician may have his or her day's surgery coordinated in one or both places.

Since opening the Pavilion, BMC is now busier than was originally projected. Obstetrics, for instance, is constantly 100 percent occupied. Baptist Medical Center again has plans on the drawing board to meet the new needs of its physicians and community. To be continually flexible and creative—this is truly the challenge of the hospital of today.

Chapter 11

Ambulatory Care
as a Survival Strategy

James A. Lamb and Susan Strong

Nestled in the Tennessee River Valley among the foothills of the Great Smoky Mountains, Erlanger Medical Center serves the industrial city of Chattanooga. Although the population of greater Chattanooga is 250,000, within a 75-mile radius 700,000 people live and work. Erlanger is a tertiary and teaching hospital affiliated with the University of Tennessee School of Medicine. In the early 1970s, however, it was a hospital in trouble.

Erlanger Medical Center, the largest hospital in southeastern Tennessee, was city-county-owned and -operated. It was, and still is, the primary provider of indigent care. Yet, the hospital enjoyed the support of private practice physicians in the community. Its facilities were decaying—the result of too many needs and too few tax dollars. Staff morale was low. Image in the community was deteriorating. Competition was accelerating.

For the hospital to survive, major changes were needed. No outpatient facilities existed. Adequate physicians' office space was not available in the area. Hospital beds and support space had to be replaced. Management concluded that if the ownership of the hospital did not change so that the hospital could do its own financing, Erlanger Medical Center would slowly die, unable to survive competition with the six or eight other hospitals in town.

Bold Action for a Dire Situation

Out of that desperate situation came a bold plan to revitalize the hospital. In 1974, after extensive planning and legislative action, the hospital's assets were transferred to an independent hospital authority. Now the hospital could issue its own revenue bonds for needed construction. With the help of an outside planning and consulting firm, a master plan for the campus was developed. Once Erlanger Medical Center issued $77 million in tax-exempt revenue bonds, the construction began.

The massive construction program included, among other things, the phased replacement of beds, a new central energy plant and laundry, a 1,200-car parking garage, and renovation and replacement of ancillary facilities. In addition, the 30-bed Willie D. Miller Eye Center, largely funded by a local foundation, was built on the campus.

As patient care facilities were being upgraded, the hospital began the development of the most visionary and far-reaching aspect of the total construction program—the physicians' office building and ambulatory care center.

Until then, little office space was located convenient to the hospital. What was available was scattered in old houses and small, privately owned buildings. Physicians' practices were unable to grow, and without growing physicians' practices, the future of the hospital looked bleak.

A consulting firm that specialized in medical office buildings and ambulatory care was retained to develop a medical staff master plan, a feasibility study, and, subsequently, a 13-floor, $14-million medical office building.

The medical staff master plan examined the primary service area and projected physician needs. It examined the hospital's medical staff and the hospital's plans for programs and services. Then, it forecast the medical manpower needed to carry out those plans and keep the hospital viable.

On the basis of this research and other market research, the consultants sized the physicians' office building. They worked with hospital management and representatives of the medical staff to detail an occupancy specialty mix that was to serve as the blueprint for leasing space to physicians.

During the process of developing the office building, the physicians were involved in the planning. Meetings were held regularly with the medical staff. Each physician was invited to meet individually with the consultants, whether or not he or she was interested in occupying the building. Many met with the consultants repeatedly.

This involvement of the physicians had two major outcomes. First, it won their cooperation and support for the project. Second, as the office building construction progressed, the physicians began seeing the project in an even broader scope. They began asking for ambulatory care facilities— separate, adequate facilities in which they could treat their outpatients. They liked the idea of having those facilities connected to the office building.

They especially wanted facilities for outpatient surgery and radiology. The facilities in the hospital were inconvenient and inadequate to handle the outpatient caseload. Hospital management saw the merits in the physicians' requests, and from this the ambulatory care center was born.

Although it might have been easy to build just a typical surgery center and outpatient radiology clinic to satisfy the physicians, management felt that bolder action was required to secure the hospital's future. As a result, hospital management, working with the board and the medical staff, decided to develop a comprehensive and visionary ambulatory care center.

As plans for the ambulatory care center developed, one more dilemma was created: how to connect it with the medical office building, now nearing completion. The solution ultimately reached was a three-story atrium that tied the two buildings together. The effect of the atrium on the project was dramatic. It created a "patient-friendly" environment that is both inviting and attractive (figure 11-1).

Step 1: The Office Building

Work began on the Medical Center Plaza office building in 1980, and it opened in 1982. The 13-floor, 159,000-square-foot office building houses physicians' offices, hotel facilities, commercial services, and some outpatient medical services. Each floor is approximately 12,500 gross square feet and 10,250 net square feet. The space is allocated as follows:

- Ground Floor: The ground floor houses extensive outpatient radiation therapy facilities, as well as a large medical oncology center.
- First Floor: Opening into the three-story atrium, this floor has commercial services and public facilities. Included are a public food service operation, private physicians' dining and meeting rooms, a retail pharmacy, post office boxes, and public toilets.
- Floors 2 and 3: These two floors consist of hotel rooms to house outpatients and families of inpatients from out of town. Each floor has 24 rooms, with 48 rooms in all. Hotel rooms are on floors with balcony corridors that open into the three-story atrium.
- Floors 4–12: These nine floors of physicians' offices house approximately 80 to 90 physicians. Each physician's office was custom-designed with standard features included in the basic lease. Optional features and more elaborate decor were added at the physicians' discretion and expense. Standard finishes included carpeting in the waiting room, vinyl floor coverings in the remainder of the office, vinyl wall coverings, window coverings, basic cabinetry and sinks, minimal laboratory space, and so forth.

As mentioned, the $14-million building was financed as a part of the $77-million bond issue. At that time, a bond issue could include up to 25 percent for projects involving individuals who would not normally be eligible to be a part of a tax-exempt issuance.

Figure 11-1.   Erlanger Medical Center, Lobby Floor Plan with Atrium

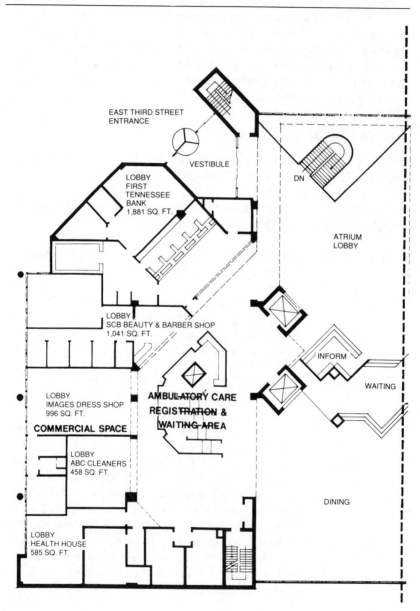

Figure 11-1. (Continued)

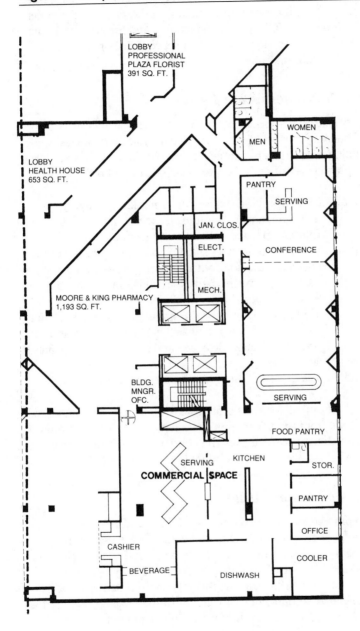

Source: Drexel Toland & Associates.

The building is hospital-owned and -operated, with physicians leasing their space. At the time it opened, the building was approximately 75 percent occupied. Today, it is fully leased. In fact, demand for office space has caused Erlanger to use two floors of shelled space in the ambulatory care center to provide additional physicians' offices.

Step 2: The Ambulatory Care Center

The ambulatory care center opened in 1983, a year after the physicians' office building. The building consists of six floors, two of which were shelled space when the building opened. As mentioned, those two floors have since been completed as physicians' offices. The floors include the following services:

- Ground Floor: This lower level houses the ambulatory surgery center and diagnostic radiology, including radiography, fluoroscopy, and CT scanning (figure 11-2).
- First Floor: This floor is at street level and opens into the three-story atrium. It includes outpatient registration and waiting areas, a branch bank, a uniform shop, and a barber/beauty shop.
- Floors 2 and 3: These two floors contain ambulatory services, including physical therapy, cardiac rehabilitation, nuclear medicine, breast cancer detection and treatment, and a clinical laboratory.
- Floors 4 and 5: The top two floors now house physicians' offices.

The cost of the ambulatory care center was $5.8 million. It was financed by investing funds from the $77-million bond issue until they were needed for construction. Interest earned over the construction life of the various projects was sufficient to pay for the ambulatory care center.

Step 3: The Connecting Atrium

In deciding to proceed with the development of a three-story atrium to connect the medical office building and ambulatory care center, hospital management considered as an alternative a one-story central lobby. However, the cost of raising the roof of the lobby to the third-story height was not much greater, and the results were significantly more functional and aesthetically pleasing. A second-floor connection to the hospital was needed anyway. Development of the three-story atrium simply facilitated that process. In addition, by raising the roof two more floors, the hotel rooms then opened onto open corridors overlooking the atrium below. Finally, the amount of height and light that the three-story atrium produced created a pleasant ambience that was much ahead of its time in medical buildings.

Figure 11-2. Erlanger Medical Center, Ground Floor Plan

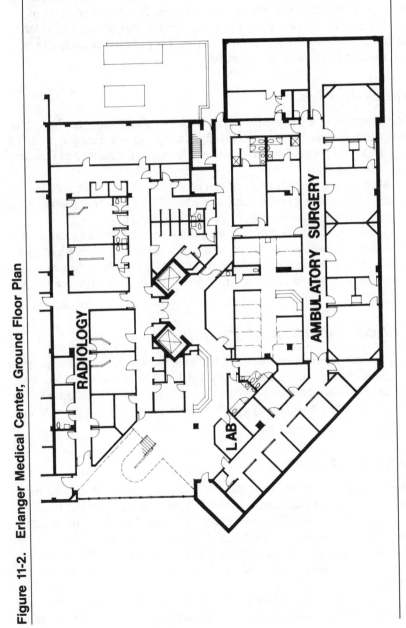

Source: Drexel Toland & Associates.

The space in the atrium is put to good use. Hotel registration is located in the center of the atrium, giving the feeling of an upscale, high-rise hotel. The surrounding area is filled with tables for public dining. It is accented with numerous plants and trees in indoor containers.

Commercial services in the two buildings are immediately adjacent to the atrium, providing a true mall-type ambience. Patients entering the office building or the ambulatory care center are directed through this central lobby area, which is attractive and unintimidating. Outpatient registration, in fact, is immediately adjacent to the atrium.

The Bottom Line

Since the completion of the project, Erlanger Medical Center has had some of the best financial years in its history. Occupancy is running at 85 to 90 percent, although that does reflect some reduction in the number of inpatient beds over the years.

Much of the hospital's success can be attributed directly to the Medical Center Plaza office building and ambulatory care center. Now bonding between the hospital and the physicians has resulted.

Currently, the office building is full, all available shelled space in the ambulatory care center has been completed as physicians' offices, and some hotel rooms are being converted into more physicians' offices. Management is now looking at the possibility of developing another office building.

Critical Elements of Planning

In retrospect, numerous elements of planning went into making this project a success. Not all of them can be discussed in this brief case study. However, two seem to have been of particular importance: first, the selection of a consultant; and second, the integration of the physicians into the planning process.

Selecting a Consultant

Once management determined that the project was worth doing and feasible, one of the next steps was to decide how to put the project together. In a large institution, staff members may have enough planning and development experience to do it themselves. If that expertise does not exist in-house or if those who have the expertise do not have the time to take on another responsibility, management will need to seek outside assistance from a consultant.

Several options are available. One is the use of a "turnkey" developer who will plan, design, and build the facility. Another option is to hire a local architect to design the building, but the result may not be as efficient or functional as desired. A third alternative is to seek the services of an experienced specialty consulting firm that can plan, design, and organize the operational aspects of the project. The consultants can coordinate the building and its program to work for the hospital within the financial parameters of the project.

In this project, Erlanger Medical Center contracted with a local architect to design the shell of the building, and an outside consulting firm was hired to plan and program the project and to work with the physicians in designing their suites.

The architects might have been able to provide services similar to those provided by the consultants. However, having experienced individuals who had designed and built numerous physicians' office buildings reduced the time required. The consultants helped the physicians decide on efficient and functional suite layouts. They also helped to mediate problems between the hospital and prospective tenants.

Including the Medical Staff

An integrated ambulatory care center and medical office building provides a great opportunity to develop a core group of supportive physicians, especially if all or part of the project can be developed as a joint venture. Input and advice from the physicians is essential, however.

No administrator, unless he or she also happens to be a physician, can order patient tests. Consequently, physician involvement is crucial to the success of the ambulatory care center and medical office building. Although it is sometimes difficult to develop the project with the physicians, it certainly is impossible to do so successfully without them. Further, with the changes in the method of capital formation, the desirability of having physicians as joint venture partners is on the increase.

Of particular importance is including those physicians who will not occupy the office building—as well as those who will—in the planning process. In this way, support is gained from both groups as they view themselves as potential users of the ambulatory care center.

One of the best ways to gain physician participation is through the formation of a Physicians' Office Building Advisory Committee (POBAC). During the Erlanger project this committee, made up of representatives of the medical staff, carried out numerous functions. For any similar project this committee could serve the following purposes:

- Provide advice on the physician mix that should be in the building
- Provide suggestions for services and programs that would best fit into an integrated ambulatory care center program
- Help establish policies and procedures for the operation of the various programs and services

- Advocate the concept to other members of the medical staff
- Help recruit needed specialists for programs and services
- Help establish the operating policies for the medical office building
- Resolve problems or disputes among tenants and between tenants and the hospital
- When joint ventures are considered, serve as a promoter of the partnership and as a source or identifier of potential investors

Certainly, other aspects of planning are equally vital to those discussed in this case study. Market research and careful planning of ambulatory care services are important. So are detailed financial planning and the development of operational methods that do not drown the center in red tape or unfairly assign hospital overhead to it.

Nonetheless, one of the most critical elements in developing this successful project at Erlanger Medical Center was getting, listening to, and acting upon good advice. That advice came from the consultants and from the medical staff. The result is that Erlanger Medical Center is no longer slowly dying. It is once again a thriving, major player in the competitive Chattanooga market.

Chapter 12

A Comprehensive Freestanding Ambulatory Care Center

Clarice V. Rech

This chapter will describe the establishment and operation of Buffalo Grove Treatment Center (BGTC), Buffalo Grove, Illinois. A brief review of how the center came to be established illustrates factors common to many ambulatory care centers.

Northwest Community Hospital is a 420-bed community hospital located in Arlington Heights, Illinois, a northwest suburb of Chicago. In 1974, an inner-city hospital proposed that a 100-bed full-service hospital be built in Wheeling, Illinois. At the time, the hospital project was not restricted to requirements of certificate of need (CON) in the state of Illinois. Consequently, the four existing hospitals in the service area joined together to oppose this effort and sponsored a study analyzing the health care needs of the area. The commissioned study showed the service area to be over-bedded, but underserved with regard to the availability of emergency care, ambulatory care, and access to primary care physicians. Ultimately, after an extended period, the proposal for the new hospital was rejected.

As a result, the existing hospitals proceeded to meet the needs defined in the study: access to emergency care, ambulatory care, and primary care physicians. In 1978–1979, Northwest Community Hospital began planning for an ambulatory care center with 24-hour emergency care to be located eight miles from the hospital in Buffalo Grove, Illinois. The Buffalo Grove area had one existing urgent care center located 1½ miles from BGTC.

After public hearings, the village of Buffalo Grove rezoned and annexed the property for the proposed treatment center. Originally, the property was farmland and zoned for agricultural use. On the property is a grove of oak trees from which the center derives a part of its name.

Demographic analysis, conducted by the hospital's executive management team, showed the population growth pattern that was projected to support the establishment of BGTC. The communities of Buffalo Grove, Wheeling, and northern Arlington Heights had a population base of 75,000 to 80,000 people, thus affording an optimal facility location, population base, and market area to be served.

The goals and objectives that Northwest Community Hospital had for BGTC—that it be a community health provider serving numerous unmet health care needs—were then satisfied. The facility opened on August 1, 1980, and became the community provider of ambulatory, emergency, and primary medical care. More than 18,000 patients were treated the first year, and full-service ambulatory care capabilities, such as X-ray and laboratory facilities, were available. The project was funded by patient-generated revenues. Construction cost $1,186,000 (excluding land costs), and expenses for capital equipment amounted to $175,500. The building has 14,173 square feet, of which 4,130 square feet are leased to a physicians' group.

An adjacent medical office building (MOB) housing physicians in multispecialty practices was established in 1982. Northwest Community Hospital now operates an X-ray and phlebotomy facility in the building, and scheduled fluoroscopy is performed there. A contract station post office was established in the MOB and operated for two years as a community service.

Factors That Affect Success

Many factors contributed to BGTC's successful repositioning to meet ambulatory care patient needs and become a carefully planned, strategically located facility. This freestanding ambulatory care facility option is one that other hospitals may wish to follow. To ensure a viable program of this nature, factors that planners must look at include market timing and market support, organizational structure and management of the facility, physical design, customer satisfaction, location, convenience, personnel and staffing, scheduling, environment for care, hospital system integration, physician components, and marketing and public relations.

Market Timing and Market Support

The timing for the establishment of BGTC was critical. The lead time prior to the opening of other facilities by competing hospitals was vital, because by the time that other facilities opened, BGTC had established its credibility and was considered the major health care provider in the community. Because of the success of BGTC, a similar facility was built by Northwest Community Hospital in 1982 in the adjacent suburban community of Schaumburg. Its success parallels that of the BGTC facility.

With regard to market support, an advisory board composed of community leaders helped determine the direction of BGTC, and various community groups have been involved since the beginning. Community involvement and support is vital.

Organizational Structure and Management

An ambulatory care center can be placed organizationally within the profit subsidiary or not-for-profit structure of an institution. Originally, BGTC was structured under the nursing department, and the managers reported to the vice-president of nursing and allied services within the hospital structure. About three years ago, the organizational structure was changed, and the treatment centers were placed under the senior vice-president.

However, the treatment center needed on-site management on a day-to-day basis, and so a treatment center manager was hired to manage all aspects of operation at Buffalo Grove. Some facilities have registered nurses who also function as business managers, but this arrangement does not always function well in practice. Laboratory and X-ray personnel at Buffalo Grove report to the treatment center manager. Technical supervision comes from the Northwest Community Hospital laboratory and radiology departments.

The responsibility for the BGTC operations rests with the manager, who is responsible for all maintenance, housekeeping, contracts, medical records, and business office functions. The manager must have the authority to hire, discipline, and release employees. The manager contributes to the revenue and expense projections and is accountable for the budget and financial decisions that are made.

The medical director of Northwest Community Hospital sets all patient care directives and oversees the physicians for the Buffalo Grove and Schaumburg treatment centers and the emergency department. The hospital contracts with a corporation of emergency physicians to provide the emergency physician staffing. Buffalo Grove Treatment Center is accredited separately from Northwest Community Hospital by the Joint Commission for Accreditation of Healthcare Organizations.

Physical Design

Buffalo Grove Treatment Center and BGMOB were designed to complement each other. The design is patterned after the physical layout and design function of the emergency department at Northwest Community Hospital and allows for the monitoring of patients from the central work station. X-ray and laboratory facilities are located conveniently for good patient flow.

Customer Satisfaction

Patient volume at BGTC has increased 8 percent a year consistently since 1980 (figure 12-1). A survey that was done by Northwest Community Hospital showed that 60 percent of the patients surveyed were return patients to the

Figure 12-1.   Patient Volume at Buffalo Grove Treatment Center, FY 1980–1981 through FY 1988–1989

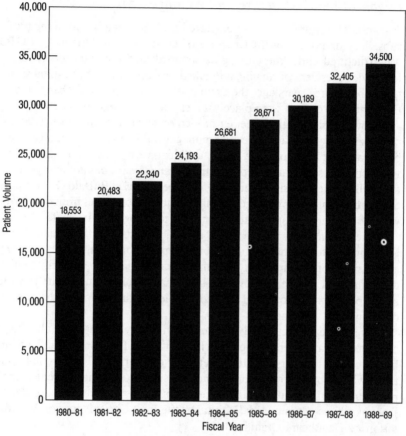

Outpatient Revenue Percent Growth

BGTC and that more than 98 percent of them would return again if an urgent care situation arose.[1] Other relevant data in the survey are listed below.

- The reasons that patients chose BGTC:
    - Close to home
    - Have been there before
    - Recommended by a friend or relative
    - Personal physician is on staff at Northwest Community Hospital
    - Close to work
    - Learned about it through direct mail
    - Recommended by physician

- What customers liked best about BGTC:
  - Caring, friendly, helpful attitude of staff
  - Prompt service and treatment
  - Efficiency and professionalism of staff
  - Location and convenience
  - Cleanliness and nice atmosphere
  - Convenient hours

Buffalo Grove Treatment Center refers patients to hospitals when necessary. Approximately 600 patients were admitted to hospitals from BGTC in 1988, and 78 percent of them were admitted to Northwest Community Hospital. After a patient's condition is stabilized, the patient is transferred either by private or fire department ambulance, depending on the seriousness of the patient's condition. Established protocols determine which mode of transportation is used.

Location

Ambulatory care centers should be located at the intersections of major highways, have easy access, and be highly visible. Buffalo Grove Treatment Center is located at the intersection of two four-lane highways, with access from both, and there is parking within close proximity to the entrances. The location is close to the major hub of activity in Buffalo Grove, and the 80-acre town center, comprising residential and retail uses, is located diagonally across the street.

Convenience

Northwest Community Hospital made a commitment to the community that BGTC would be open 24 hours a day, and the treatment center's signage reflects that availability. At least one physician is on the premises at all times, with overlap coverage during periods of peak volume.

Personnel and Staffing

Staff members of BGTC are very customer-service-oriented and are aware of the customer relations aspects of their jobs. The receptionist at the front desk, who greets the patient, sets the tone for the patient's entire experience at the facility. All staff members are flexible and work as a team, performing such multitask functions as admitting, discharging, and accepting payment at the time of service. The majority of the staff has been with the BGTC for the past seven years, which provides both continuity and conformance. All personnel are certified in cardiopulmonary resuscitation.

The registered nurses (RNs) have varied backgrounds but must have a minimum of three years' experience, preferably in a critical care area. All must have proficiency in intravenous and cardiac monitoring, and half are currently certified trauma nurses. The radiological technologists (RTs), who are trained as generalists, are registered and have a minimum of one year's experience. The BGMOB RTs also do phlebotomy and specimen gathering. Secretaries are skilled in computer use and in public relations. Staffing of the facility is according to hours of operation and days of the week and is illustrated in table 12-1.

Scheduling

A constant analysis of trend lines at BGTC is done every month to determine high volume and its impact. Summer is the time of highest volume; the months with daylight saving time have the heaviest volume in the afternoon and evening, whereas during standard time, the heaviest volume is during the day shift. From May to October, an additional staff person (a nurse) is assigned to the 5 p.m.-to-8 p.m. time period to assist with the volume and to help cover staff mealtimes.

Recent trend lines on Sunday evenings showed the necessity of additional secretarial hours, which were approved. Last year, the laboratory trend lines demonstrated the necessity of additional start-up time for the laboratory machinery, as well as an increase in laboratory tests performed, and so an additional hour of staffing was added. Flexible personnel hours, staffing, and the use of on-call personnel are vital to the smooth functioning of BGTC. The BGMOB RT and the BGTC RT fill in for each other at lunchtime.

The employees' commitment to this smooth functioning was demonstrated when an on-call registered nurse developed a schedule for employees who volunteered to be on call at certain hours to assist the night nurse with the increasing work load. It is normally difficult in health care to attract personnel willing to perform on-call duties when required. Employee volunteers are an important component of the BGTC staff, and the center would have difficulty functioning without their consistent support.

It is crucial to have enough on-call nursing personnel to be able to fill in on short notice, and all staff members have been flexible in this regard. Monitoring of trend lines and volume indicators shows that the heaviest volume days are, in order: Monday, Wednesday, Tuesday and Thursday (equal), Saturday, Sunday, and Friday. The registration process should flow on a 2:1 ratio (2 admissions processed for each discharge), so that smooth flow is maintained.

Summer help, such as medical students, is hired for secretarial positions. Registered nurses are the most flexible staff members, because they can perform phlebotomy, but they also command a higher salary. Buffalo

Table 12-1. Staffing Coverage, Buffalo Grove Treatment Center and Buffalo Grove Medical Office Building

Buffalo Grove Treatment Center (BGTC)

Service	FTE	Days	PMs	Nights
X-ray	2.8	7:30 a.m.–4:00 p.m.	4:00 p.m.–12:30 a.m.	12:30 a.m.–7:30 a.m. (Call)
Lab	2.6	7:30 a.m.–4:00 p.m.	3:30 p.m.–11:00 p.m.	Specimens sent to Northwest Community Hospital lab
RN (includes RN who also is the manager)	6.55[a]	7:00 a.m.–3:30 p.m.[b] 8:00 a.m.–4:30 p.m.[b]	3:00 p.m.–11:30 p.m.[b] 4:00 p.m.–10:00 p.m.[b]	11:00 p.m.–7:30 a.m.
Janitorial	1.0			10:30 p.m.–7:00 a.m. Weekend coverage by contract
Secretary	1.9[a]	9:00 a.m.–3:30 p.m. weekdays 10:00 a.m.–6:30 p.m. weekends	3:30 p.m.–10:00 p.m. weekdays	

Buffalo Grove Medical Office Building (BGMOB)

Service	FTE	Days	PMs	Nights
BGMOB RT	1.0	8:30 a.m.–5:00 p.m. weekdays		
Physician coverage		7:00 a.m.–5:00 p.m.	3:00 p.m.–11:00 p.m.	9:00 p.m.–7:00 a.m.

[a] To be increased.

[b] Schedules are separate for separate "swing" or overlapping purposes (for example, to accommodate patients at end of shifts).

Grove Treatment Center relies mainly on its own staff to fill in during heavy volume because of the specialized nature of the work.

Cash reconciling and bank depositing are done during the registered nurse overlap between 3:00 and 3:30 p.m. and also during the night by the night registered nurse.

Environment for Care

The ambience that is created by the BGTC staff and facility is vital. The staff is professional, pleasant, efficient, and thorough. The staff role is to be the patient's advocate with a "high-touch/high-tech" approach where patients feel that the staff cares about them in an environment that provides the latest in high-technology medical equipment. Follow-up is provided through the referral physician call roster, and patients are instructed according to their disposition and treatment with their physician. Immaculate cleanliness of the facility is maintained to produce the right environment for care.

Hospital System Integration

The establishment of BGTC affected all departments within the Northwest Community Hospital system, and a period of adjustment was required for everyone to become acclimated to the requirements of this new facility. Figure 12-2 illustrates how the day-to-day operations essential to the smooth running of BGTC are performed by both BGTC and Northwest Community Hospital.

Physician Components

Approximately one-third of the patients seen at BGTC have attending physicians on staff at Northwest Community Hospital, one-third have attending physicians not on staff, and one-third have no attending physician at all. Patients without an attending physician are referred for follow-up care to the appropriate physician on call. Physicians in each specialty take rotating call for the treatment centers and emergency department.

From the outset, BGTC worked with the attending physicians. Patients are not referred to physicians in BGMOB except at their specific request. Routine physical examinations are not done at BGTC.

Marketing and Public Relations

The key to the success of BGTC has been word-of-mouth advertising by satisfied consumers. The credible name of Northwest Community Hospital has also been an important factor. The public relations department of Northwest Community Hospital includes BGTC in its annual and monthly publicity.

Figure 12-2.   Day-to-Day Operations at Buffalo Grove Treatment Center

Supplies:	A courier service delivers supplies to BGTC four days a week.
Radiology:	Radiologists review all X-ray films daily. Transcription is done at Northwest Community Hospital, and reports are returned to BGTC.
Laboratory:	Both the chief pathologist and the laboratory manager at Northwest Community Hospital provide technical direction to BGTC. The supervisors of hematology, chemistry, and microbiology routinely visit and inspect the BGTC lab for compliance with Northwest Community Hospital policies and procedures. The majority of laboratory tests are done at BGTC. The remainder are performed at Northwest Community Hospital.
Electrocardiography (ECG):	A new computerized ECG system allows the ECGs to be transmitted to Northwest Community Hospital for interpretation and returned with the diagnosis.
Medical Records:	Medical records are stored onsite. After six months, they are microfilmed and retained at Northwest Community Hospital.
Business Office:	Approximately one-third of the patients pay at the time of service. Major credit cards are accepted. The patient is given a copy of the bill at the time of service, but computerized billing is sent from Northwest Community Hospital.
Pharmacy:	Supplies are delivered by courier and transported in a locked container.
Education:	Staff members can avail themselves of ongoing educational programs at Northwest Community Hospital. Community education programs are provided to the community free of charge on an ongoing basis. Instructors are provided through the Continuing Education Department.
Dietary:	Limited special dietary items for patients and staff are delivered by courier. Special-occasion meals are provided for the staff of BGTC, similar to those provided to other Northwest Community Hospital employees.
Marketing and Public Relations:	Buffalo Grove Treatment Center is included in hospitalwide programs. At times, special literature and communications on BGTC are distributed.
Engineering:	Equipment safety checks are performed onsite by the biomedical engineering staff.
Housekeeping:	Initially, housekeeping services were by contract. This year, the addition of a staff person to perform housekeeping services five nights a week was approved. Services on weekends are still by contract.

Some advertising is placed in local publications. For the past several years, BGTC has staffed the first-aid station for Buffalo Grove Days, a special community event, thereby generating positive publicity among the target audience.

Blood pressure screening on a walk-in basis was done as a community service but had to be curtailed to between 2 p.m. and 4 p.m. daily, when additional staff is available. Callbacks are done two days after the patient's visit to determine satisfaction and to answer questions regarding follow-up care.

Productivity and Profitability

Although patient volume has increased since 1980, BGTC's full-time equivalent (FTE) allocation has not increased proportionately. The approved FTEs increased from 12.6 for fiscal year 1980–1981 to 17.97 for fiscal year 1988–1989. Figure 12-3 shows that the FTE allocation has been exceeded, but because the coverage is monitored on a pay-period basis, it has kept in balance with the volume service required. The number of patients versus the productive hours gives a productivity monitor factor, as shown in the following formula:

$$\frac{\text{Total Productive Hours/Pay Period}}{\text{Total Patients/Pay Period}} = \text{Productivity Monitor Factor}$$

The productivity factor goal is 1.0 to 1.1.

The highest generation of volume and correlating revenue produces the greatest revenue if cost can be minimized. Payment at the time of service is encouraged; the amount of bad debt is decreased if some payment is made at the time of service. The patient record has a portion allocated to the billing-payment function, which simplifies submission to third-party payers.

Special System Improvisations

At BGTC, the patient record was developed as all-inclusive to serve multiple purposes and eliminate duplication of efforts. Laboratory and X-ray requisitions form a part of the record, which can easily be detached to order and charge the patient simultaneously.

Telephone outpatient laboratory orders are written on simple order forms and filed at the reception desk to facilitate quick registration. X-ray release folders and release cards are kept at the front desk for simplified release and pick-up. The X-ray file system is color-coded for ease in finding X-ray folders and identifying those that are misfiled and out of sequence.

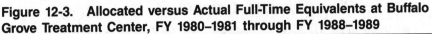

Figure 12-3. Allocated versus Actual Full-Time Equivalents at Buffalo Grove Treatment Center, FY 1980–1981 through FY 1988–1989

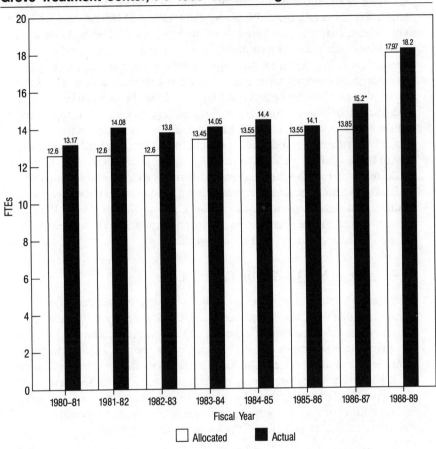

*Addition of 1.0 FTE housekeeper

The computerized ECG system has an automatic copy feature so that copies can be made immediately should the patient require admission. Statistical logs are maintained at the time the patient record comes off the printer, which eliminates confusion and delays during times of heavy volume.

Inventory control of supplies is monitored on a constant basis, and a three-year master accounting system was developed to compare expenses. Routine monitoring of this information is conducted in order to avoid collecting additional data when questions arise. Assignments for routine duties are shared by various staff members.

Future Planning and Growth

Originally, BGTC thought that volume would level off at 25,000 patients per year. However, the estimated volume for 1988–1989 is 34,500 patients, and all signs indicate that continued growth will be experienced. The facility and its function were designed for a volume of 25,000 patients per year, and the continued increase has begun to challenge available resources, including space.

Additional space requirements include more registration and discharge areas so that patients can be processed faster and their privacy can be ensured. Also, the original area designed for X-ray storage has been outgrown, and additional space will have to be found. Additional space also is needed for medical record storage, and a better system for keeping medical records will have to be devised. In addition to fulfilling space requirements and improving the medical records system, several other issues are important in planning for BGTC's future. The first two, maintaining the quality of patient care and retaining and recruiting staff, concern the ongoing effectiveness of BGTC's operations, whereas the issues of new growth and expansion will prepare BGTC for the services consumers will require in the future.

Maintaining the Quality of Patient Care

With regard to maintaining the quality of patient care, the commitment to high-technology services will continue at BGTC. However, acquiring and operating these services is becoming more difficult as volumes continue to increase and quick patient turnaround time becomes of the essence. Having the treatment center manager perform two functions, that of manager and staff member, is becoming increasingly more difficult in practice. Another factor that affects patients' perceptions of the quality of care is length of waiting time. Patient waiting times are beginning to increase slightly, and this will eventually affect patient satisfaction if the increases are not contained.

Retention and Recruitment of Professional Staff

The BGTC staff has a high morale that must be maintained. The nationwide shortage of registered nurses will affect BGTC at some point. An esprit de corps was established in the beginning, and efforts must be made to keep the professional staff that has served so well. Most of the personnel live in the community, and new personnel are usually recommended by current employees. It is important to listen and act upon suggestions or complaints when possible.

New Programs

Buffalo Grove Treatment Center serves as the health center for the community. The community room, which can seat 50 persons, is used by various health-related organizations, such as weight-reduction groups, Alcoholics Anonymous, Cocaine Anonymous, domestic violence support groups, head trauma support groups, and support groups for parents of children with malignancies.

Buffalo Grove Treatment Center can continue to build on its existing programs, such as industrial programs and contracts that can be tied in with Northwest Community Hospital. These programs should encompass workers' compensation, wellness, and education, as well as employment physicals coordinated with attending physicians. In recent years, Northwest Community Hospital has developed a corporate health program, which encompasses many of these new programs.

Women's health and physical fitness programs and facilities are becoming more prevalent and could be implemented as additional services. Special testing, such as audiometry, could be added, and mammography could be performed at BGMOB. In addition, as the community health center for the community, BGTC could dispense home care and durable medical products.

Expansion

The community of Buffalo Grove is continuing to grow and to become more developed. The town center has 300 units for senior citizen housing and includes other residential, retail, and commercial uses. Expansion to keep pace with increased volumes will be required, and planning has begun to resolve space restrictions. The restraint of having only one X-ray examination room, for example, will have to be addressed.

As volume continues to increase, long-term additional facilities in the hospital's service area may be required to meet patient care needs. An example of this kind of facility diversification is Palatine Family Health Center, located in Palatine, Illinois, midway between the treatment centers in Buffalo Grove and Schaumburg. Established in 1986 by Northwest Community Hospital, it operates more as a family practice and primary care facility and is open 12 hours per day, from 8 a.m. to 8 p.m. Although placement of this additional facility in the general service area can affect patient volumes at both facilities, it is too early to assess the impact that Palatine Family Health Center has had on patient volume at BGTC.

It is possible that other facilities may be added by other groups or hospitals as the ambulatory care market continues to grow. It is important to determine ongoing community health care needs and to provide them.

In the July–August 1987 edition of *Chicago Consumer,* Northwest Community Hospital's BGTC was rated number one in patient visits in the Chicago metropolitan area.[2] The intention is to continue to build on this success, to create strategies and facilities to provide the services consumers will require in the future, and to accomplish this in the most cost-effective manner possible. Thus, Northwest Community Hospital is facing a unique opportunity to further expand the availability of ambulatory care services in new market areas.

References

1. Northwest Community Hospital. *Six Month Survey.* Arlington Heights, IL: NWCH, 1986.

2. White, O. R. Chicago's top hospitals. *Chicago Consumer.* July–Aug. 1987.

Chapter 13

New Construction and Reorganization of Ambulatory Care Services

William J. Graham

As the 1980s began, Penrose Health System, a 460-bed not-for-profit hospital system that operates Penrose Hospital and Penrose Community Hospital, occupied an enviable position among health care providers in Colorado Springs, Colorado, and surrounding El Paso County. (Penrose Health System is now Penrose-St. Francis Healthcare System effective with the merger of these two facilities in 1987.) It stood as the dominant provider of acute care medical services in the area. Its flagship institution, Penrose Hospital, was considered the elite hospital in terms of the quality of its attending medical staff. It had created outstanding, widely recognized treatment programs for cancer, heart disease, and other serious illnesses. It was firmly rooted in the history of its city. Its admissions were growing each year, as was the city's population, and occupancy consistently exceeded 85 percent. Penrose seemed secure in its role as the health care leader in the Colorado Springs area.

Yet Penrose had its inadequacies. Its physical facility was aging; the newest addition to the hospital was in 1959. Overburdened operating rooms caused difficulties in scheduling. Space was at a premium, and that which existed was inefficient and overused. Many services, especially outpatient programs, were scattered in a disorganized fashion throughout the facility, cramped into inadequate quarters. Entering the hospital was both confusing and inconvenient for everyone—patients, visitors, physicians, and staff. The result was not only poorly used and inadequate space but also an unattractive and institutional appearance.

Outpatient services were viewed by Penrose, as by most hospitals, as complementary offerings to inpatient care rather than important sources of revenue and patient contact in their own right. Revenue generated by outpatient programs accounted for 11 to 13 percent of the hospital's total

revenues, a not insignificant amount, but not of primary importance. Inpatient care remained the primary function and primary area of concentration of Penrose Hospital.

Changes in the Health Care Environment

Soon after the decade began, the health care industry experienced one of the
most dramatic changes in its history: Medicare instituted its new prospective
payment, or diagnosis-related group (DRG) system, with its far stricter regulations for reimbursement for services, its emphasis on shorter inpatient stays,
and its consequent encouragement of greater use of outpatient services in an
effort to contain costs. Other third-party payers began to follow suit. The traditional hospital's primary business — inpatient care — was threatened. Penrose
experienced the same effects that were felt throughout the health care industry: declining admissions and average daily census, shortened lengths of stay,
and increasing expenses with little or no growth in patient revenues. Medical-
surgical admissions at the main hospital, which had been steadily rising,
dropped sharply from 14,800 in 1981 to approximately 13,500 in 1982. Penrose
faced the realization that its most important market was shrinking.

At about the same time, Penrose's management recognized that the
hospital's market leadership position was, and indeed had been, eroding.
An analysis of statistics revealed that although the area's population was
growing at approximately three times the national average, admissions to
Penrose had been growing at a slower rate even before the DRG system went
into effect. Total surgical procedures performed were declining despite a growing outpatient surgery program. The utilization of other outpatient services
was also dropping. Although the market for traditional hospital services
was without a doubt declining, the inescapable conclusion was that Penrose was losing market share both in inpatient admissions and in outpatient
services.

As Penrose was losing market share, other institutions were gaining it.
In Colorado Springs, as in most of the nation, health care institutions were
altering their perceptions of the ethics of marketing and advertising and
were undertaking aggressive promotional efforts to attract patients to their
institutions and practices.

Under the pressures of increased competition, hospitals were searching
for new kinds of services to offer, new ways to deliver traditional services,
new methods of controlling costs while maintaining a high quality of care,
and new ways of communicating their messages to patients. Penrose had
to undertake that search as well to retain its market dominance and then
regain its market share.

The first step in successfully designing services to appeal to the patient
was to recognize the emergence of a new kind of health care consumer: the

convenience customer. As women, who make the majority of health care decisions, entered the work force in increasing numbers in the 1970s and 1980s, the need for new, more cost-effective and convenient health care delivery systems became acute. More and more patients now seemed to put convenience on a par with high quality in their criteria for selecting health care providers. This new convenience customer, in combination with financial incentives and restrictions that encouraged the use of outpatient services, exerted powerful pressure on the health care industry to change its systems and methods for delivering services. Penrose realized that it faced competition not only from other hospitals, but also from freestanding emergency and surgery centers.

Physicians were also feeling the effects of increased competition. Historically, Colorado Springs has always had a surplus of physicians, with a supply that was 10 to 15 percent higher than national ratios. The advent of the convenience customer created even more intensive competition among physicians in a market already oversupplied with health care providers. Part of their response to the competitive atmosphere was to join new types of health care organizations: health maintenance organizations and preferred provider organizations. By 1982, approximately 20 percent of the civilian population of Colorado Springs, which has a substantial military presence, had enrolled in one of these new health care plans, and the percentage was almost certain to grow. Penrose recognized that these organizations would increase the pressure to find different, less expensive ways of delivering high-quality medical care and that outpatient services would play a key role in those new delivery systems.

Strategies for the 1980s

If no one expected the sweeping changes in health care that the decade of the 1980s brought, no one could long avoid recognizing the extent of the challenges facing hospitals and physicians and the need for new strategies. To survive, much less succeed, Penrose would have to reassess many of its long-held assumptions, reinterpret existing trends from a new perspective, and identify opportunities for developing new services. With projections indicating that inpatient admissions would continue to decrease, or at best remain level, Penrose realized that outpatient services would become critical to its financial health and growth. In addition, Penrose recognized the importance of outpatient programs as entry points for patients into the health care system.

An initial review indicated that all the outpatient programs and services identified as important to health care consumers already existed in the Penrose Hospital facilities: emergency services, day surgery, laboratory and blood bank, diagnostic cardiology, pulmonary medicine, radiology, nuclear medicine and ultrasound, and rehabilitation services. The primary problem Penrose faced was in making services more accessible, cost-effective, and convenient to patients by providing adequate and appropriate space for them and in making the outpatient service areas, including registration, more attractive and efficient.

In addition, however, Penrose recognized that the convenience customer was increasingly likely to use freestanding ambulatory care centers for basic family and minor emergency care. In 1982, the first of such centers opened in the Colorado Springs area. Penrose determined that its own best interests and those of its attending staff would be served if the hospital entered this new field rather than allowing a competing institution or organization to take the initiative in filling the need for ambulatory care.

These conclusions spurred Penrose to undertake two major building efforts in the early 1980s: the creation of a network of ReadyCare Centers offering general medical care and minor emergency treatment, and the construction of a new, full-service ambulatory care center at the hospital itself.

ReadyCare Centers

The attending staff initially viewed the ReadyCare Centers as an attempt by Penrose to directly compete for primary care patients with its own physicians. The main challenge that Penrose faced was to build cooperation between the hospital's management and its medical staff to ensure the success of this network of health care centers. Penrose had to clarify to the medical staff its key objective for the ReadyCare Centers: to provide convenient points of entry into the health care system for new patients, who could be referred to the attending staff for continuing care and who would use Penrose for outpatient and inpatient care.

This goal of creating cooperation was advanced when Penrose, along with a committee of medical staff members, created operational guidelines for the ReadyCare Centers that ensured attending family practitioners that they would, in fact, directly benefit from the centers. Physicians practicing at the ReadyCare Centers are hired directly by Penrose, rather than participating in joint ventures, and they do not have admission privileges to the hospital. Patients requiring continuing care or admission are referred to a member of the Penrose attending staff.

The policies and practices of ReadyCare, which have been proved over time to the attending staff, have resulted in building trust that allows an attending physician to refer his or her own patients to ReadyCare for treatment when the physician is not immediately available. The attending staff has learned that they will not lose their patients permanently to the Ready-Care network and that they will benefit from the continuing referrals from ReadyCare to their practices. Penrose carefully tracks and reports those referrals and monitors the practices of each ReadyCare Center to ensure the effectiveness of the network in bringing patients to Penrose and to its attending staff.

Ambulatory Care Center

In constructing its new ambulatory care center (ACC), Penrose faced less medical staff resistance but greater financial and organizational challenges. Until recently, hospitals in Colorado were required to obtain certificate-of-need (CON) approval in order to make substantial alterations or undertake new construction. The state agency responsible for approving CON applications was resistant to any hospital construction at that time, and plans for several hospital projects were repeatedly reviewed by the agency. Ultimately, the agency did not approve that portion of the ACC plan that called for the construction of three dedicated outpatient operating suites in the new ambulatory care center. This necessitated scaling down the proposed building from four stories with 25,000 square feet each and a basement to three stories and a basement. Approval to proceed was obtained, however, and construction on the three-story addition began in late 1982. Residents of the area immediately surrounding the hospital had some objections to the construction project, and this resistance delayed the approval process for several months as the hospital and community leaders discussed their issues.

The primary objective in building the new center was to facilitate the entry of patients into the Penrose Health System by offering convenient, high-quality services that would enhance the hospital's image and bring those patients back to Penrose for inpatient treatment. Also important was maximizing the cost-effectiveness of outpatient services in order to build ambulatory care services into a more important source of direct revenues.

The key design objectives for the reorganization of the ambulatory care areas were to maximize access and convenience; to create a clear, separate vehicular access and a distinct pedestrian entrance; to deinstitutionalize the space and make it more attractive and welcoming and less clinically intimidating; and to enable Penrose to convert existing space easily and to expand in the future without additional major construction and renovation. The project also made it possible for Penrose to improve overall access to the hospital for patients, visitors, physicians, and staff and to improve the hospital's general convenience and appearance.

In designing the new ACC, substantial attention was given to patient convenience and flow, particularly with regard to the distance from the registration desk to the various service areas and the number of turns the patient would need to make to locate the desired area. Priority was also given to providing convenient access from the ACC on every level to the existing Penrose facility to ease staff flow and the use of ancillary services by inpatients. The plan was to also provide easy access from the ACC to campus-based physicians' offices and other hospital services. Two important consumer services—the Women's Life Center, which provides information, referral, and educational programs on women's health issues, and the Professional (retail) Pharmacy—were incorporated into the first floor of an attractive two-story atrium that connects the ACC with the hospital.

To select locations for the various outpatient services in the new building, Penrose studied projected patterns of utilization as well as space requirements to determine which services should be located together to maximize patient flow and convenience. Almost half of the first floor of the building was dedicated to an easily accessible, open, and attractive outpatient registration and waiting area.

An area for laboratory sample collection and radiology services was conveniently located no more than 75 feet from the registration area. A separate storefront entrance on the atrium mall provides a beautifully decorated and private reception area for the Breast Diagnostic Center.

In addition, a substantial portion of the first floor is used for a new emergency department with greatly improved vehicular and pedestrian access. Space initially reserved for meetings and educational activities has now been converted into a rehabilitation center with its own entrance. This center is designed especially for the outpatient who requires nonintensive therapy.

The second floor houses an expanded and greatly improved nuclear medicine and ultrasound department, the histology laboratory, the blood bank, and the Cardiology Center, which provides diagnostic cardiology and rehabilitative services. This arrangement was selected to make access to all these key services as convenient as possible for patients requiring comprehensive laboratory services and for cardiac patients, who are likely to require blood studies and nuclear medicine diagnostic services as well as the specific services of the Cardiology Center. The second floor also allows easy access to the main hospital's surgical suites through a connecting corridor for outpatient surgery patients.

The third floor contains most of the ACC's rehabilitative services and is designed to serve inpatients who require physical and occupational therapy as well as outpatients who need lengthy and intensive therapy sessions. The Respiratory Therapy Center is also located on this level.

The basement of the ACC houses meeting rooms; the training and education area; a comprehensive wellness program that includes weight control, stress management, and other preventive health care services; personnel offices; and space for future expansion of rehabilitation services.

The new ACC was designed and built to provide maximum flexibility for reorganizing the interior space. Expanding or reducing the space allotted to a particular service area or creating space for a new area without having to undertake new construction is relatively simple and inexpensive.

The Results of Change

Since the new ACC opened in late 1984, Penrose has experienced substantial growth in outpatient service utilization. This growth confirms the accuracy of Penrose's original projections and the need for the full four stories of space called for in its initial plans. New outpatient surgery suites and an improved staging area for outpatient surgery patients are being added on the second floor in an area adjacent to the existing operating room and proximal to ACC services.

Outpatient visits for 1987, not including visits to the emergency department, numbered more than 124,000, an increase of 51 percent from a low of 82,000 just before the ACC's opening. Annual outpatient registrations (that is, number of individuals served) are up by more than 20 percent, from approximately 30,000 in 1984 to nearly 37,000 in 1987. Outpatient surgery continues to grow despite the lack of dedicated facilities for this service; 53 percent of all surgical procedures performed at Penrose in 1987 were performed on an outpatient basis, in contrast to 1982, when 17 percent of all hospital surgeries were outpatient. The improved and expanded facilities in rehabilitation services have led to more than a fourfold increase in outpatient rehabilitation visits since 1985. Rehabilitation services have indeed been the shining star in overall growth, accounting for more than half of the total increase in visits.

Overall, inpatient utilization has also improved at Penrose. Although the total number of surgeries performed at Penrose continued to decrease during the period from 1982 through 1984, the increasing popularity of outpatient surgery has led to an overall increase in surgeries for the past three years. As a result, Penrose has regained its dominant position in surgery procedures, with a growing market share of these procedures done in the hospitals.

Inpatient utilization of rehabilitation services has almost doubled since 1984. Finally, although medical-surgical admissions remain significantly lower today than during the period prior to 1982, the average length of stay increased from 7.5 to approximately 8.3 days. This increase is indicative of the case mix intensity; that is, fewer but sicker patients remaining in the hospital setting.

In 1987, Penrose outpatient revenues equaled 20 percent of the hospital's total revenue, as compared to less than 12 percent in 1982. Although outpatient revenues may not represent the greatest contributions to the hospital's total revenue, the services delivered to outpatients are likely to be less cost-intensive and therefore more profitable than are many inpatient services. The criterion of percentage of revenue is unlikely to reveal the most important information that hospitals need to evaluate the real financial contribution of outpatient services.

Even more significant, perhaps, are the figures indicating that the amount of revenue per outpatient visit has increased from approximately

$125 prior to 1980 to $450 as of 1987. In addition, the number of outpatient visits per patient has increased from 2.7 in 1980 to 3.5 in 1987. Penrose has found that different types of management information systems and data collection are necessary to accurately monitor the outpatient business.

Statistics also indicate that outpatient services are delivered to three or four times more patients than are inpatient services in any given year. The additional opportunities to interact with patients and physicians, to provide them with high-quality service and positive experiences, and to market other services are substantially higher than in inpatient care. The vital necessity of establishing and maintaining a service orientation in providing outpatient services cannot be questioned. Patients not only want high-quality medical care; they also want high-quality service in its delivery.

Convenience, ease of access and patient flow, and attractive surroundings in outpatient service areas are critical to that service orientation. Of even greater importance is the leadership of the hospital in setting a strong, clear, and consistent course toward improved consumer service. No ACC, no matter how well conceived, well intentioned, or well designed, can succeed without the complete dedication of the hospital's management and its leadership in setting goals and objectives for outpatient programs. A strong consumer orientation in outpatient service may well be the deciding factor in the patient's selection of a hospital, not only for outpatient care but also for inpatient care.

Chapter 14

A Medical Mall Prototype

Sister Elise Boudreaux and Patrick W. Philbin

Providence Hospital, part of Providence Medical Center, is located in Mobile, Alabama, and has a rich history of service to the community. This Daughters of Charity hospital began in very humble surroundings in downtown Mobile, and grew to represent one of the major health care providers. In the mid-1960s, the hospital's proportion of government-sponsored and indigent patients began to increase, and by the 1970s Providence began to experience some problems such as declining utilization. Most health care providers in Mobile were located in the downtown area, with the majority of hospitals and almost all physicians located within a two-mile radius. In the 1980s, Providence reviewed its position, looked toward the future, and decided to relocate to the growth area eight miles west of downtown.

Planning and Developing the New Providence

The hospital administration and staff went through much anguish during the process of obtaining certificate-of-need (CON) approval, because the relocation would absent them from the downtown area. The move was predicated upon the changing population and the fact that the majority of all hospitals were located in the downtown area. It was important to reestablish Providence as a health care leader and reemphasize its philosophy and mission of service.

During the phases of strategic planning and seeking CON approval, it became obvious that the hospital's design had not kept up with the changing and volatile health care marketplace. Between the time of the initial decision to move the hospital and the time of the actual construction, major changes had come about in the health care industry. There was a movement to alternative systems of care and a deemphasis of the inpatient hospital. In addition, ambulatory care became much more important, as utilization of inpatient facilities declined both in number of admissions per 1,000 people in the population and in average length of stay. Declining utilization equates with decreased revenues, a problem experienced by many hospitals in the country. Providence was caught in the changes both in focus and in delivery of health care. Another concern was that although the proposed hospital was architecturally attractive and modern in comparison with the old facility, physicians were not necessarily attracted to the new site, because their medical practices resided almost totally in the downtown area.

The Next Steps: Design and Staffing

A consultant was brought in to begin working with the hospital to look at the issues of physician mix and balance. Studies were performed to determine the potential needs of the new service area population, as well as the mix and balance of physicians most appropriate to the new hospital site. There was a total review of the original concept and design of the traditional hospital site, with a bold move to develop an integrated, futuristic health campus.

This proposed health campus emphasized alternative delivery and integration of service options. The design focused on needs and demands of the population, as well as on improved efficiency and productivity for physicians. These issues were becoming more and more important in a competitive marketplace as physicians nationwide, especially those in metropolitan areas, began to realize the increasing marketplace pressures. The proposed health campus focused on how health care would be delivered in the future. The inpatient hospital remained the backbone of the campus, but was no longer the only focal point. Research into the behavior of consumers and the use of shopping centers uncovered the high concern for convenience, cost-effectiveness, attractiveness, and continuity of care. It became apparent that people who used inpatient services actually preferred alternatives to inpatient care and wanted options in the way in which care was delivered.

The new site was expanded to incorporate an ambulatory care center (referred to as a vertical hospital) for ambulatory patients, which housed physicians' offices, ambulatory care programs, shopping facilities for patients, radiation therapy, ambulatory surgery, and a diagnostic center. The ambulatory care center emphasized ease of access, convenience, cost-effectiveness, efficiency, and attractiveness. The proposed center for the ambulatory patient would stand side by side with the traditional inpatient hospital, which was designed for the bed or litter patient. In addition, the campus included future sites for centers for substance abuse, mental health, rehabilitation, and various stages of elderly housing and care.

The consultant also developed a basic mix and balance of physicians that would be necessary to contribute to the growth of the new campus. Various corporate and organizational structures were considered, as well as joint ventures with the physicians. It became apparent that heavy involvement and participation of the physicians was essential to the success of the new Providence. Extensive interviews were held with providers to test the new health campus model and refine important issues in relation to the campus.

The concept of the new Providence, a dramatic change in model design and delivery, was calculated to also change the practice patterns of the physicians and draw them to the organization as a preferred place to practice. A master site plan, with a focus on the health care campus, was taken to the medical community in an effort to negotiate a move from the downtown area to the new site. There would be 122 physicians assigned to practice at the new health care campus. The physicians, upon reviewing the changes in the industry and in Mobile, took on the risks that went with becoming a part of a new, convenient, efficient, and integrated model of health care delivery. They found a win/win situation with relation both to their patients and to their individual practices.

The New Providence: Step by Step

In the heat of battle it is seldom obvious that logical steps are being followed to reach the decision to move forward. The logic will vary from case to case, based on the pressures and priorities being faced by that organization. In the case of the new Providence, the following steps were used in planning and building the health care campus:

1. The hospital recognized the need for change. At this step there was a series of events, related both to finance and to utilization, that called into question the viability of the present hospital. There were continual changes in medical staff utilization, and it was obvious that other hospitals were being used as alternatives to Providence Hospital. The downtown area continued to reflect a stable-to-declining population, with more of the population moving to the west. Through assessment of the utilization, the revenues, and the socioeconomic conditions in Mobile, it became apparent that there was a need for change. On the basis of this realization, three options were developed: (1) remain at the present site; (2) move various components of the facility; or (3) move the entire health care operation. The advantages and disadvantages of each were explored.

Option: Stay
Advantage: Less disruptive
Disadvantages: Continued declining resources and utilization; poten-
                tial insolvency

Option: Move part of operation
Advantages: Retention of existing operation while developing new
                operation
Disadvantages: Prohibitive cost, less efficiency

Option: Move total operation
Advantages: Gain new presence; growing marketplace more con-
                venient to patients
Disadvantages: Disruptive; difficult risks

2. Once the advantages and disadvantages of each option were explored,
   the third option was chosen: to move the entire operation. The hospital studied the health care delivery system and the population to see
   where the greatest opportunities existed. A study was made to decide
   where the population was moving in the Mobile metropolitan area.
   The study reaffirmed suspicions that much of the population was
   moving to the west of downtown. This population included many
   of the new immigrants to the Mobile area as well as the general middle class. After in-depth research it became obvious that a move of
   somewhere in the vicinity of eight miles to the west on a major
   thoroughfare would be an excellent strategy for Providence Hospital.

3. The hospital began planning to move to a new site. Different strategies were considered to find which was most appropriate to moving
   to the new site. At that time, CON was an important component
   of planning for the future, so the hospital needed to incorporate the
   regional and state health care criteria to gain approval for the move.
   Questions about whether there should be a gradual phasing in of
   the development or whether a total move would be the best option
   were continually addressed.

4. The hospital assessed the current marketplace in relation to physician practice patterns. Cursory reviews revealed that physicians continued to have traditional practices in the downtown area, but with
   the major concerns about preparing for the CON process, they actually reduced their energy and effort in this particular arena.

5. The hospital reviewed the changes in health care nationally and
   regionally. In the case of Providence, the traditional inpatient, cost-
   plus, sellers' market was still in existence. Changes nationally and
   regionally actually came about after approvals had been finally given
   and building had commenced. At that time, there were few indications that major change was occurring in the health care industry.
   Regionally there was consistent conservatism in the way in which

medicine was practiced and health care was provided. There was little change anticipated in many of these elements other than technological improvements.
6. The hospital designed an overall strategy to provide high-quality, cost-effective, convenient, and attractive health care. To this end, two options were considered for the new campus: (1) continue to emphasize the traditional hospital focus; or (2) emphasize a new concept emphasizing ambulatory care.

Option: Traditional hospital
Advantages: Highest comfort and knowledge
Disadvantages: Continued reduction in use; less attractive to physicians; higher risk

Option: New campus focusing on ambulatory care
Advantages: Trend-setting; attractive; convenient; efficient
Disadvantages: Higher risk that accompanies new developments; more difficult to accomplish

After much thought and discussion, the ambulatory care campus concept was selected. Although the initial design was more traditional, the redesign took into account the new buyers' market, which demanded much more sensitivity to the public in relation to convenience, as well as cost-effective, high-quality care. The redesign that occurred at this point focused on the future of health care delivery and regained a strong position in the marketplace by incorporating the newest ideas into the overall design of the health campus and the ambulatory care center.

7. The hospital evaluated its corporate and organizational structures. When designing the strategy it is important to be able to put the organization in the most flexible posture for providing services. If alternative services will be developed, and if there will be some areas of competition or conflict as well as the opportunities for joint venture, the organization must be structured to allow these different activities to occur without dramatically inhibiting one another. Much in the way that big business uses corporate structures as a means to control both liability and operational variance, the health care industry must also use and perhaps redesign organizational and corporate structures. Seldom do traditional structures resolve the problems of a hospital when rapid changes are required and the issues are many and complex.

8. The hospital obtained the necessary approvals to move the campus. The majority of all approvals had been gained through prior activity to obtain CON approval, and in this stage of revision it was only necessary to go for minor changes to complete the CON process.

9. The hospital predicted and reviewed inpatient and outpatient volumes by analyzing current conditions and looking to the future. It was

necessary to predict potential volumes to allow financial feasibility studies to be performed. The area in which it was most difficult for Providence to predict volumes was ambulatory care. This generally is true because the methodologies used to predict volumes in the inpatient area are different from those used in the outpatient area of health care. Also, there are almost no available or accurate data on outpatient care to predict future utilization.

10. The hospital phased in the development in relation to priorities. That is, it took the most important components and worked them through to establish a good foundation and then phased in the development of the different parts of the campus. It is important to introduce each phase at the proper time, based on its order of priority. If there is an attempt to do too much too fast, the result can be tremendous confusion. If, on the other hand, movement is too slow, the window of opportunity may be closed by the time the effort has been achieved. It was obvious that the inpatient and ambulatory centers were most important to this campus development.

11. The hospital reviewed the projections for needed medical staff. Achieving the proper mix and balance of medical staff for the new health campus was essential. If, for example, there are too many physicians for one specialty, that can create an imbalance in relation to the rest of the physicians on campus. The goal is to have a target number for all specialties in the recruitment program.

12. The hospital developed a schematic (three-dimensional) model of the campus development and especially the physicians' offices. This allowed the medical staff to visualize their new offices.

13. The hospital developed a specific strategy for negotiating with physicians for office space that used professional selling and closing methods. The ground rules and framework for negotiation must be developed in advance to allow logic and consistency to prevail throughout the negotiating process.

14. The hospital began negotiations with physicians. The opportunities available to them with the new health campus and the various arrangements through which they could be achieved were presented. Even though physicians were involved in many of the developmental issues, this was the time for very specific negotiations. These negotiations should center on the needs of the patients, the physicians, and the corporate structure and policies of the hospital or system. During this period, development can begin with those components that have the support of the user group.

15. The hospital opened the facility. In many cases this will be a phased opening, with major components opening jointly. The entire campus probably will open much in the way that a shopping center

does, with major anchor facilities made available to customers while the other components are still being negotiated. The new Providence Hospital and the ambulatory center were opened simultaneously in the summer of 1988.

Conclusion

The example shown by the new Providence Hospital illustrates that a hospital caught in the changing health care delivery marketplace can position itself to deal with these changes and successfully develop an attractive, efficient health care campus. Much faith, preparation, risk, and effort were required from the hospital community. However, the outcome is that the new campus is open and gaining strength every day in providing sensitive, high-quality, caring, efficient, cost-effective, "new era" care to the people of Mobile.

Chapter 15

Ambulatory Care Expansion in a Community Hospital

Kenneth J. Natzke and Patrick W. Philbin

St. Joseph Medical Center in Bloomington, Illinois, has been a leading provider of health care to area residents for several decades. The orientation of the hospital has been to provide inpatient care and to work with the medical community to see that patients receive the best quality of service with cost-effective charges. As the health care industry began to change from an inpatient to an alternative, outpatient orientation, St. Joseph found itself in a less competitive and less attractive situation, especially in relation to physicians.

The new thrust toward ambulatory care created several new challenges. Physicians began to develop freestanding ambulatory services that competed with the hospital. Other large hospital providers set up satellite clinics in the Bloomington/Normal area to provide health maintenance organization (HMO) services and some primary care to feed their tertiary facilities.

Originally there were three competing hospitals in the community. Two of those hospitals merged, effective July 1, 1984, putting St. Joseph in a much more competitive situation than before. St. Joseph began to lose some market share to this new merged competitor. Physicians received attractive offers from the new competitor for both office space and practice alternatives. A review of the utilization trends reflected that although at one time St. Joseph had been very strong, its position in the marketplace was continuing to weaken. Dramatic change was necessary if the Sisters of the Third Order of St. Francis, who managed the hospital, were to retain their presence in the community.

Planning for Change

A consultant was employed to help the hospital review alternatives, develop options, and plan for change. Historic as well as competitive marketplace data were used to analyze the changing marketplace and inpatient patterns of use at the hospital. Medical staff were surveyed to ascertain changing practice patterns and to gain a more complete understanding of the Bloomington/ Normal market. The dramatic move to alternatives, particularly ambulatory care, was a major thrust in the community. It was important to the physicians to improve productivity and revenues through improved use of their time and through investment in entrepreneurial ventures.

Part of the challenge was to consider some changes in the existing corporate structure of St. Joseph to allow new ways to organize and protect the assets of the hospital. Physicians were migrating to the new merged hospital system because of special alternatives that the new competitor had available to them.

After several weeks of analysis and deliberation, a plan was adopted to enhance the existing campus with an ambulatory center, or "vertical hospital" for ambulatory patients. The center would house physicians' offices and ambulatory services and treatment and would place St. Joseph in the forefront of health care delivery. The ambulatory center was designed to accommodate many of the concerns of the physicians and to provide an alternative to inpatient care that would be a win/win situation for both the hospital and the physicians. The development of this ambulatory care center was based on the knowledge that there needed to be enough synergism and availability of services to attract both physicians and the general public to the facility.

In essence, the vertical hospital centralizes ambulatory services in one location — the traditional hospital's health care campus — rather than fragmenting ambulatory health care into various independent freestanding facilities and services. The best location for a vertical hospital generally is on the health care campus adjacent to the traditional hospital. Patients who need immediate transfer benefit from the proximity. The backup of the traditional hospital is an advantage to continuity of care because it allows physicians to use alternative delivery modes with the knowledge that acute care services can be made available immediately.

The operational and functional design of the vertical hospital can be specific to each component, such as ambulatory surgery, diagnostic testing, and so forth. Components can also include ambulatory home care, rehabilitation, and monitoring of chronically ill patients. In some cases, the vertical hospital will be the home base for satellite outreach services.

The obvious outcome of the vertical hospital is the centralization and integration of alternative health care services. This effort achieves the priorities of continuity of care, cost containment, patient convenience, and program viability.

The Timing of the Change

The timing of the change was crucial, because with long-term deliberation and bureaucratic red tape, decisions could have been prolonged much past the patience of the interested physicians. Many of those in the medical community were preparing to develop competing freestanding centers. It was because St. Joseph realized the critical nature of the decision and the need for immediate decisive action that it was able to move into the marketplace in a positive manner and develop the vertical hospital without heavy costs that can result from long-term deliberations. The windows of opportunity were very small and needed almost immediate action. On the other hand, they also needed to be thoroughly investigated to make sure that the opportunity was real and the return on investment to both the patients and the organization was adequate.

Without movement in this new area, there would have been continued deterioration of physician utilization at St. Joseph. The medical community realized that change was necessary, and that if they showed enough commitment, they could become a part of that new direction. The Sisters of the Order had a more fundamental question: whether or not they could continue their presence in the Bloomington marketplace. Once this decision was renewed, St. Joseph's plans to fully enter the ambulatory marketplace became necessary.

Often a medical office building is relabeled or renamed an ambulatory center, but does not actually contain the additional components necessary for a true ambulatory center. In developing the concept of the vertical hospital, it was taken into account that small strip shopping centers had significantly less attraction and draw for consumers than the larger, more comprehensive shopping centers. The same is true for an ambulatory center: although the backbone is the availability of physicians, additional services are essential to provide both continuity of care and a continuum of care. People are looking for a one-stop shop; otherwise they will be forced to move from one fragmented, freestanding center to the next, which results in a great deal of inconvenience and inefficiency for patients and physicians alike.

In St. Joseph's case, the hospital and the Order responded to the needs of the community, to the physicians, and to the demands for ambulatory care with an attractive and efficient design to house the ambulatory components that were most appropriate for this community. Physicians who were in the process of developing a series of freestanding, fragmented ambulatory centers were able to stop and consider St. Joseph as an alternative. They realized that it would be much more efficient and much more attractive to patients and to themselves to have a comprehensive center that incorporated all the different services necessary. It was through this kind of logic and reasoning that the ambulatory center was developed. It is making a dramatic impact on the position of St. Joseph in the marketplace.

The Steps Used in Planning

The steps used to accomplish the changes at St. Joseph can be used by any health care organization to plan a program that meets the needs of both the medical staff and the community to be served. These steps are as follows:

1. *Recognize that a commitment to the reorganization of ambulatory care is a top priority.* In many cases there is a realization that both utilization and revenues are declining without an acceptance that this trend is real and will continue. Some administrators, boards, and physicians confuse their hopes with realities. There have been two fundamental changes in the industry: the change from a sellers' to a buyers' market, and the change from a cost-plus to a competitive pricing market.

2. *Decide whether it is necessary to bring in outside expertise to complete the assessment, or whether internal expertise can carry out the analysis.* The use of consultants adds financial responsibility to the organization. It is important to realize that operational issues demand the full time of the existing administrative and management team, and it is more cost-effective to use consultants who will concentrate specifically on areas needing full-time, immediate attention. Once the decision about using consultants is made, a specific plan of action is necessary. The decision should be based upon availability of people, their commitment and full dedication to the assessment, and their ability to present objectively the outcome of the investigation.

3. *Select the appropriate people to perform the analysis.* Whether selecting a consultant or internal staff to perform the analysis, it is critical to select people with both the ability and the time to assess the problems. Often administrative interns or finance people are assigned the problem of assessing a strategic planning or marketing issue. This is neither appropriate nor in the best interests of the project. It is essential to use experts to perform the analysis.

4. *Develop an action or work program with specific timetables for conducting the analysis.* It is important to develop a work program so that the results of the analysis will have a specific due date. Also, providing key decision makers with the action steps and interim reports is very useful in helping people understand the progression of the analysis.

5. *Develop recommendations.* Recommendations must be made in relation to both the analysis of the situation and the organization within which potential changes must occur. At times, recommendations are made that are totally out of step with the mission, philosophy, and direction of the organization. In this case, little will be accomplished. It is important to develop recommendations that mesh with the organization's mission, goals, and objectives, or to recommend changes in these areas prior to making the recommendations.

6. *Develop an internal consensus with all relevant parties.* Once the administrative group has accepted the recommendations and the direction suggested by those recommendations, it is important to review or monitor that direction in relation to the parent organization and the physicians, all of whom will be significantly affected.

7. *Perform a financial feasibility study to ensure the solvency and financial potential of the recommendations and the specific components.* In some cases, even though the overall direction shows financial solvency, some of the suggested components do not have the necessary volumes to break even. At that point it becomes an administrative decision either to provide the service because of need or to discontinue its provision until volumes can be increased.

8. *Develop an implementation plan.* An implementation plan must be developed and will differ from hospital to hospital and from situation to situation over time. An implementation plan must include acceptance by and commitment from the significant actors. Joint ventures must be designed, developed, and approved through the organization or its parent, as well as from legal and financial perspectives. The implementation plan should include a schedule to ensure that the necessary changes are accomplished in an acceptable time frame. In the case of St. Joseph, there was heavy commitment on the part of the administrative team, once it received approval from the parent corporation, to move swiftly to negotiate with physicians and develop the necessary commitments for the ambulatory center.

The New St. Joseph Ambulatory Center

The design components of the ambulatory center took into consideration the same driving forces that attract people to shopping centers. Components of convenience, cost-effectiveness, efficiency, variety of options, and attractiveness were all addressed in the design of the new center, which opened in September 1989 (see figure 15-1).

The involved physicians have been very supportive of the ambulatory center. Because many of them were involved in the initial planning, the ambulatory center reflects much of their input. More important, the new center enables them to offer their patients more options for their health care needs. These are among the many benefits that resulted from the planning of the St. Joseph ambulatory center.

Figure 15-1. Eastland Medical Plaza

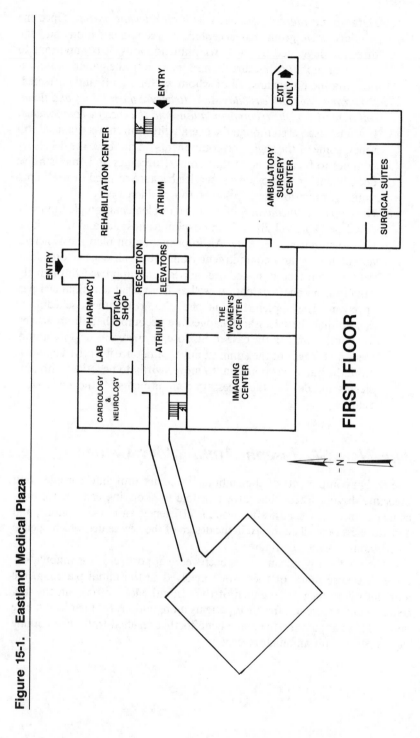

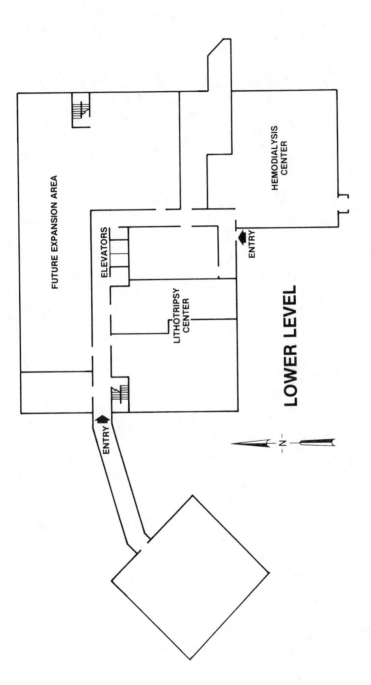

FUTURE EXPANSION AREA

ELEVATORS

LITHOTRIPSY CENTER

HEMODIALYSIS CENTER

ENTRY

ENTRY

LOWER LEVEL

N

Source: Patrick Philbin & Associates, Inc.

Chapter 16

A Full-Service Ambulatory Care Center and Physicians' Office Building

James A. Lamb and Susan Strong

Washoe Medical Center in Reno, Nevada, is the primary tertiary hospital in the sparsely populated northwestern Nevada and northeastern California area. Reno itself has a resident population of approximately 150,000. The hospital's total primary service area, which encompasses a 200-mile radius, includes about 650,000 people.

As a tertiary hospital, Washoe is the center for several regional programs, including open-heart surgery, cancer treatment, rehabilitation, and renal dialysis. It is also a teaching affiliate of the University of Nevada School of Medicine. Although licensed for 512 beds, it is currently operating approximately 350, with renovation projects under way.

When the administration of Washoe Medical Center changed hands in 1983, plans were already under way for a freestanding cancer treatment center. It was to be located on a narrow strip of land on the west side of the hospital campus.

Aware of the growing trend toward outpatient care, the new administration began to evaluate the hospital's lack of ambulatory care services and facilities. What they saw was a need for more outpatient diagnostic capability, expanded dialysis, and same-day surgery.

However, the natural direction for expansion of ambulatory services was on the east side of the hospital campus, where more land was available. Locating new outpatient facilities on the opposite side of the campus from the cancer treatment center made little sense. Having ambulatory services scattered from one end of the campus to the other would be cumbersome, inconvenient, and inefficient. Consequently, plans for the cancer treatment center were put on hold while management took time to reconsider.

What emerged from further discussion was a plan for a more comprehensive ambulatory care center. It would include the cancer treatment center as well as a dialysis center and same-day surgery services. All would be housed in one building on the east side of the campus.

As planning was proceeding for the ambulatory care center, hospital management also began to see a need for a physicians' office building. Although many office buildings were located around the hospital, the hospital had no control over their occupancy. When physicians moved out, they were not necessarily replaced by other physicians. In addition, a new office building was being planned near the hospital. As physicians began looking at the proposed building, a number of them came to management and asked, "Can't the hospital provide us with a better alternative?" The physicians wanted to be near the planned ambulatory care center.

At this point, Washoe Medical Center contracted with the consulting firm of Drexel Toland & Associates of Memphis, Tennessee, to conduct a feasibility study for an office building. They did an in-depth analysis of the medical staff and the office market. They found that many of the buildings in the area were old and poorly maintained. Many physicians wanted to expand their practices and were looking for a place to move. Other physicians had expiring leases and wanted new space.

The preliminary study showed that an ambulatory care center with an attached physicians' office building would be well received. Only one other major hurdle had to be cleared before the project could proceed.

At the same time that the preliminary planning was taking place for the ambulatory care center and physicians' office building, Washoe Medical Center was in the midst of a major reorganization. Until November 1985, the hospital was owned by the county. At that time its assets were transferred to a not-for-profit corporation.

The parent corporation, Washoe Health System, Inc., now operates the hospital, a foundation, a health maintenance organization (HMO), and a network of outlying hospitals. In addition, a number of for-profit subsidiaries have been formed to operate the commercial laboratory, home health program, nursing home, durable medical supply company, and private-duty nursing program.

With organizational restructuring complete, Washoe Medical Center was ready to proceed with the development and construction of its office building, ambulatory care center, and the final element, a two-level parking garage. The consultants were retained to program and design the physicians' office building and its ambulatory and commercial areas. A local architect was hired to complete design of the ambulatory care center.

The Physicians' Office Building

Although the ambulatory care center had been the first segment of the total project to be planned, construction of the physicians' office building, The

Washoe Professional Center, began first. It got under way in 1986, with the first tenants moving into the building in the fall of 1988.

The consultants programmed and sized the office building based on the medical staff master plan and marketing studies they had done. In addition, they relied on input from hospital management and the physicians. The resulting office building was designed with eleven floors and 195,290 square feet of space. About 43,000 square feet is net rentable commercial and ambulatory care space. In addition, the building includes two floors of hotel and outpatient guest rooms. Total cost for the project was approximately $23 million.

Space in the building is utilized as follows (see figures 16-1 and 16-2):

- *Ground floor.* The ground floor is used exclusively for ambulatory care services. Located on this floor are a central admitting and waiting area for outpatients; a multipurpose clinic; a wellness center with exercise room, sauna, steam room, lockers, showers, and dressing area; an imaging center, including magnetic resonance imaging (MRI) and computed tomography (CT); counseling rooms, conference rooms, and classrooms; a laboratory drawing station; and rooms for physical therapy, occupational therapy, and communication disorders.
- *First floor.* The first floor is allocated for commercial services. Included are a pharmacy with a durable medical equipment showroom, a uniform and apparel shop, a dry cleaner, a hair-styling shop, a gift shop, a video rental store, an automatic teller machine, a restaurant and deli, and private dining and conference room facilities. In addition, this floor includes an information and guest check-in area and mailboxes for building tenants.
- *Floors 2 and 3.* The second and third floors comprise 48 hotel or guest rooms, with 24 rooms on each floor. The corner rooms on each floor have small kitchens and can be made into suites. Because Washoe Medical Center serves a large geographic area, this arrangement is especially helpful to families of out-of-town patients. In addition, each floor includes a conference room for guest use.
- *Floors 4 through 10.* These seven floors of physicians' offices were designed to accommodate about 70 physicians. When construction was started, about half of the space was committed. By the time the building was completed, all space was filled, with physicians continuing to call to inquire about space.

The Washoe Professional Center design incorporated state-of-the-art technology. All floors were wired into the hospital's central computer system. Hardware and software were carefully researched for the physicians and recommendations were made to them for the most effective systems for their offices.

Figure 16-1. Washoe Professional Center, Ground Floor

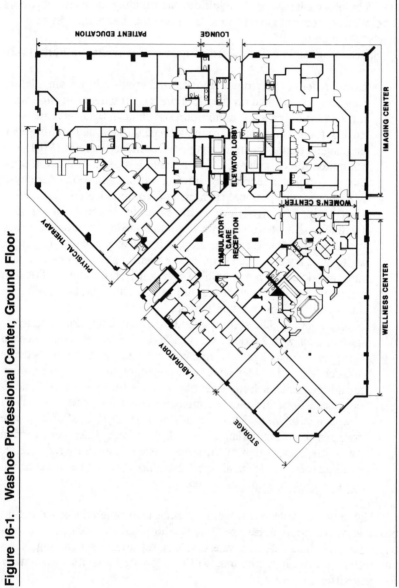

Source: Drexel Toland & Associates.

Figure 16-2. Washoe Professional Center, First Floor

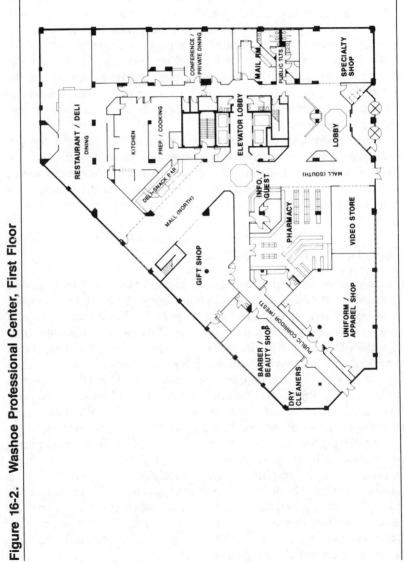

Source: Drexel Toland & Associates.

If they choose, physicians may use computer systems that will tie into the hospital's system, which gives them access to the hospital's clinical management system. Such access enables physicians to admit patients, update inpatient medical records, handle billing, and perform a number of other functions without ever leaving their offices. In addition, every physician's office is equipped with a direct telephone line to the hospital to make handling all types of arrangements more convenient.

In a building that incorporates such a variety of uses as ambulatory care, hotel and guest rooms, and physicians' offices, security is always a problem. Again, computers have been used to develop a refined system to meet all needs. Magnetic cards are issued to physicians for use in entering the parking lot, entering the building after hours, and operating the elevator after hours. During nonbusiness hours, elevators operate only to the floors to which they are keyed in this manner. Thus, hotel guests can get into the garage, the building, to their floors, and into their rooms, but they are unable to take the elevators to physicians' office floors, for example, except during business hours.

Another advantage of this system is that through the central computer, the hospital can tell at any time which physicians are parked in the garage or if they have entered the building. In an emergency, the system speeds up the process of locating the physician. Security is further enhanced by a television surveillance system that is monitored by hospital security.

The Ambulatory Care Center

The ambulatory care center was constructed as a two-story building, with the structural capability to expand to four floors. The building consists of 60,558 square feet. Total project cost came to $10.8 million.

The ambulatory care center is positioned closer to the hospital than is the office building tower. This facilitates the use of the center by inpatients when necessary. Although it is designed for outpatient use, approximately 10 percent of the dialysis patients, for example, are inpatients. Other inpatients may use the cancer treatment center or the MRI and CT scanning capabilities of the imaging center in the office building. For that reason, the ambulatory care center and those ambulatory care services in the office building that are used by inpatients are located with maximum convenience to the hospital. Both the ambulatory care center and the office building are connected to the hospital by enclosed corridors at two levels. One is a public connection. The other is for physicians and inpatients traveling back and forth between the facilities. When inpatients are brought to the ambulatory care facilities, they travel a minimum distance. This arrangement protects them from having to be wheeled through public areas. It also minimizes the exposure of ambulatory patients to inpatients.

The ground floor of the ambulatory care center connects directly to the ground floor of the office building. Thus, this whole level in both buildings is used for ambulatory services. The entire ground floor of the ambulatory care center is dedicated to cancer treatment. It includes radiation therapy, radiation physics, the Northern Nevada Cancer Council, the statewide tumor registry, and other support services. The first floor includes a large renal dialysis center and shelled space for a same-day surgery unit.

Both the ambulatory care center and the office building are positioned so that one side of each opens onto a triangular courtyard. The courtyard is landscaped with shrubbery and small trees and is equipped with outdoor furniture. It not only provides a pleasant view from both buildings, but it also offers a cheerful outdoor spot for employees or patients to relax during a break or at lunch.

The Parking Garage

The third element of this total construction program was a 450-space, two-level parking garage. It is located adjacent to the office building and the hospital. Built at a cost of $2 million, the garage provides parking for physicians and emergency room patients on the ground level.

The upper level, structured similar to an airport drop-off zone, provides a circular drive with loading and unloading areas for the office building, ambulatory care center, and hospital. The center section of the upper level is used for visitor parking and patient admitting.

The Financing Package

Financing for the physicians' office building and parking garage was arranged through a master lease program with Merrill Lynch. Merrill Lynch holds the title to the building in escrow and has it financed through commercial paper. Washoe Professional Center, Inc., a for-profit subsidiary of Washoe Health System, Inc., master-leases back the building and garage.

The financing arrangement was based not on construction costs, but on the appraised value of the facilities, or on the cash flow projected for a fully occupied building. Because of that arrangement, Washoe was able to receive 100 percent financing. In fact, the total project cost for the office building ($23 million) and the garage ($2 million) came to $25 million, and the appraised value upon which financing was obtained was $26 million. Thus, a nice cushion was obtained for handling any operating losses that might occur during the start-up phases of the project.

This financing package was very complicated and took eight months to arrange. Under this scheme, new financing will have to be arranged in five years or the building will have to be bought back from Merrill Lynch. The current financing does have a major advantage, however. It removed the debt from the hospital's books. This particular type of financing is no longer possible because of changes in financial accounting standards. At the time it was arranged, however, it met the specific needs of the hospital.

The ambulatory care center was financed separately and much more traditionally. It is owned outright by Washoe Medical Center, Inc., and was financed through tax-exempt bonds.

Ambulatory Care Planning Issues

One of the major decisions to be made in planning an ambulatory care center is determining who will operate the services being offered. The decision-making process is complex and requires much thought.

If hospital departments are to operate the services, several hurdles must be cleared. One of the first objections management may encounter is that personnel may not want to relocate part of their department to an outpatient center. Operating from one location is much easier for them. They may be inclined to let the patient find them, rather than take their service to the patient. Unfortunately, in the hospital industry, decisions are sometimes made on the basis of convenience to employees, rather than convenience to the patients.

Another hurdle is that splitting departments between inpatient and outpatient areas may not be the most efficient method of providing a service. However, dollars generated from new outpatient programs may well offset any perceived loss of efficiency. In fact, if management can stimulate personnel to think more broadly, they may find that organizing separate inpatient and outpatient service areas can actually bring an expansion of service capabilities.

To decide whether or not various hospital departments should operate the specific outpatient services in Washoe's ambulatory care center and physicians' office building, management asked several questions. What are the organizational capabilities of the department heads? Are they capable of running a service that is oriented to outpatients? Will they attempt to organize it in the same manner as the inpatient program?

Outpatient care in an ambulatory care setting is oriented to fast, efficient, convenient care. At the same time, the care must be of high quality and must be delivered in a sensitive manner. Too often, department heads are not accustomed to thinking in these terms. They are used to having the patient in a "captured" state as an inpatient—subject to their scheduling system. At Washoe, management decided that its department heads did have the flexibility and vision to develop and manage the outpatient programs.

In situations where the right combination of circumstances and personnel do not exist, administrators might want to look at the following alternatives:

1. *Leasing.* Because of a desire or need to find alternative sources of capital for a given service, hospital management may find that leasing the proposed ambulatory service could be the best alternative. The hospital may not have the financial resources to budget for a hospital department to operate both an inpatient and an outpatient service.

   Leasing can be a positive direction to take if the institution does not have the time, talent, or resources to develop the service adequately. The hospital may share in the profits of such a venture through the lease income as well as through a percentage of gross or net revenues.

2. *Joint venture.* Because of the desire to generate support from a physician or group of physicians, hospital management may want to consider joint venturing a particular service. Risk sharing is becoming an increasingly popular vehicle whereby physicians and hospitals develop ambulatory care services.

3. *Contract management.* Contract management is still another alternative to a hospital department providing an ambulatory service. Although this arrangement is similar to leasing, it can provide the hospital with more financial control over the service.

Conclusion

The Washoe Ambulatory Care Center and Professional Center is successful because several goals were established. First, the hospital wanted to be able to satisfy third-party payers, who are increasingly demanding ambulatory care services. Second, hospital management wanted to provide in one location a convenient vehicle for diagnosis and treatment for all outpatients as well as the patients of building tenants. Third, management wanted to strengthen its bonds with the physicians. Fourth, management wanted to develop a level of trust and confidence with its medical staff that is not possible with off-campus offices.

If short-term approval is any forecast of long-range success, the goals at Washoe are being met and will continue to be met through its ambulatory care and physicians' office center. Such success is no accident, however. It requires thorough study and careful planning. It also requires cooperation among the hospital management, the hospital board, the department heads, and the medical staff. Finally, it requires skilled implementation by experienced professionals. Today's health care market is no place for timid players. The success at Washoe and at other hospitals depends on acting upon, not just thinking about, current trends and market demands.

Chapter 17

Ambulatory Care in an Academic Medical Center

Ellen Marszalek-Gaucher

The University of Michigan Medical Center (UMMC), located in Ann Arbor, Michigan, is one of the oldest and largest academic medical centers in the country. The hospital was established in 1869 to serve as the core teaching facility for the University of Michigan Medical School. By the 1960s, the medical center complex had grown to include 1,000 beds located in 5 hospitals and more than 100 specialty clinics providing care to 305,000 outpatients per year.

In 1970, anticipating major changes as a result of such environmental factors as competition, changes in physician supply, shifts in referral patterns, and an antiquated adult hospital facility built in 1925, the administration of the hospital and the university regents made the decision to begin planning a replacement hospital facility that would include 888 adult medical-surgical beds, a complete range of diagnostic and therapeutic services, and the specialty clinics. The final project would cover more than 1 million square feet and cost $210 million.

At first, the Michigan Department of Public Health, through its federally designated planning agency, the Comprehensive Health Planning Council-Southeast Michigan (CHPC-SEM), refused to give its approval because health care planning guidelines indicated that southeastern Michigan already had too many hospital beds. Many people argued against the new facility. However, the argument that the medical center was an important resource for the entire state prevailed, and the certificate of need (CON) for the full project was granted in September 1979.

Concurrent with the planning for a new facility was the need to review UMMC's ambulatory care programs, which were in dire need of reorganization and consolidation. Over the years, these programs had been scattered in a variety of buildings, making systems support difficult, if not impossible. Just delivering the medical records for clinic visits was a monumental effort. The provision of services had become expensive and oriented toward providers rather than toward consumers. The general demeanor of the facilities was drab and unfriendly, and the facilities were not easily accessible to patients. Much planning would be needed to create the types of services offered by private physicians in the community.

During the certificate-of-need review, the ambulatory care portion of the project became a political football. In the late 1970s and early 1980s, debate centered on whether ambulatory care should be included in the project. Budget problems loomed as a major hurdle for the ambulatory care space as it became apparent that the budget would not cover all planned parts of the project. The Project Review Committee of CHPC-SEM recommended not approving the ambulatory care facility. However, the governor of Michigan, William Milliken, who was a progressive thinker, approved the project and advised the university that his approval was contingent on an ambulatory care component. He believed that in an era of increased national growth in ambulatory care, the medical center could hardly afford to build a premier health care facility without provisions for this important, growing segment of the health care business. In August 1981, an amended CON was approved, and work began on what was to be called the A. Alfred Taubman Health Care Center.

When the decision was made to include the ambulatory care component, an accelerated planning process was instituted to help this segment of the plan catch up with the rest of the project planning. A committee of administrators, physicians, and planners was selected to review other new ambulatory care facilities in the country and to select an architectural firm. A series of visits was planned to new ambulatory care facilities.[1] Committee members reviewed design features and operational efficiencies or systems that supported care. The visits helped to identify the features that UMMC wished to have, as well as some problems it could avoid.

The shape and size of the building was constrained by the size of the site, a problematic small, rectangular, footprint-like area that required an architectural solution. A curved, cantilevered portico two stories high was designed to be built over the driveway to expand the assignable space without expanding the rectangular space. The overhang would provide shelter from the elements as well as needed additional space for faculty offices. To provide the necessary 300,000 square feet of space, which was projected based on the needs of the project, the building had to be four stories high. Fortunately, most of the original planning for the hospital building had been completed before the project was put on hold, and hence data from the ambulatory care market survey were available for review. The market survey focused on existing programs and current market penetration, projected volumes, educational requirements, the influence of research on space requirements, review of management and operating policies, and, finally, an estimation of total space needs. This study was used as a baseline measure.

Planning the Project

One of the first steps in planning the ambulatory care facility was to create an inventory of current space and a description of patient visits to obtain a profile of services. Each hospital department chairman was interviewed to determine new program opportunities, assess the transition from inpatient to outpatient care in each area, and indicate any new technology on the horizon that should be included in the plans. An external consultant, using computers, analyzed and evaluated the results of the interviews.

A prior study, completed in 1979 to facilitate a cost-effective approach to examination room utilization, was used to plan changes to existing facilities.[2] The hypothesis established for the utilization study was that significant improvement in patient turnaround times would reduce the number of examination and treatment rooms needed and would thereby reduce project or construction costs. The study indicated that the center would need to achieve an average rate of 36 minutes per patient visit, rather than the 75-minute patient rate suggested in a previous study. The average time in the examination room plus a 15-minute period between patients plus the number of patients seen per year plus projected visits and the projected number of examination rooms available in 1990 yielded a module allocation for each department (table 17-1).

Implementing the Plans

A group called the Ambulatory Planning Committee met concurrently with the hospital's planning committee to complete the planning process. A revision of the institutional mission statement was conducted, and from this an Ambulatory Care Mission Statement was drafted. The mission statement emphasized an environment of excellence:

- Ambulatory Care Services has as its primary mission the creation of an environment where excellence in patient care services is paramount. We believe an environment of excellence is filled with compassion for those who come for care; a commitment to the highest standards of clinical service; a continual search for new knowledge; leadership in preparing future generations of health care professionals; and an environment that encourages employee participation in effective problem resolution.
- To this end, Ambulatory Care Services' overall direction is for the planning, development, coordination, and monitoring necessary to provide superior-quality, cost-effective outpatient services in response to the needs of the citizens of Michigan and the surrounding states.

A definition of ambulatory care was also devised to ensure institutional agreement with the definition and plans. Schematic designs were developed

Table 17-1. Assignment of Examination Room Modules Using Average Time in Examination Rooms, University of Michigan Medical Center

	I Average Time (Min.) in Exam. Rooms[a]	II Average Time in Exam. Room Plus 15 Min. between Patients	III Patients/Year/ Exam. Rooms[b]	IV Projected Visits in 1990s[c]	V Number of Exam. Rooms in 1990s[c]	VI Number of Modules in 1990	VII Adjusted Allocation of Modules in 1990s[d]	VIII Resultant Allocation of Exam. Rooms (VII x 8)	IX Ratio of Exam. Room Allocation to Exam. Room Need (VIII:V)
Dermatology	32	47	2,553	16,700	6.5	1.0	1.0	8	1.2
Employee health	—	—	—	6,500	—	0.5	0.5	4	
Internal medicine	66	81	1,481	61,300	41.4	5.5	6.0	48	1.2
Neurology	48	63	1,904	10,900	5.7	1.0	1.0	8	1.4
Otolaryngology	31	46	2,609	26,200	10.0	1.5	1.5	12	1.2
Surgery	38	53	2,264	55,900	24.7	3.5	4.0	32	1.3

[a]Source is Clinic Time Study.
[b]Assume 250 days per year, 480 minutes per day, or 120,000 minutes per year.
[c]From paper on outpatient volumes, January 5, 1982.
[d]Extra modules are distributed to the departments of internal medicine and surgery because of the internal allocation within each department to the various subspecialty services.

that characterized ambulatory care services, consisting of the specialty clinics, the emergency services, the transportation system, helicopters, ambulances, and the satellite (A. Alfred Taubman Health Care Center), as a funnel to channel patients to inpatient and ancillary services. Subsequently, a planning model was devised, as well as a list of significant issues to be discussed during the planning process. These issues included the following:

- Protect and expand market
- Develop a primary care feeder system
- Forge strong working relationships with institutions to lead to networking
- Enhance clinical services to stress convenience, access, and price
- Protect financial viability
- Implement strong financial development program
- Downsize the expense base
- Build the revenue base

These were issues used for major presentations to administrators, physicians, nurses, and support staff to discuss the planning goals and objectives. Figures 17-1 and 17-2 show the planning steps and the planning model presented in the discussions.

Figure 17-1. Steps in the Planning Process for Ambulatory Care Development, University of Michigan Medical Center

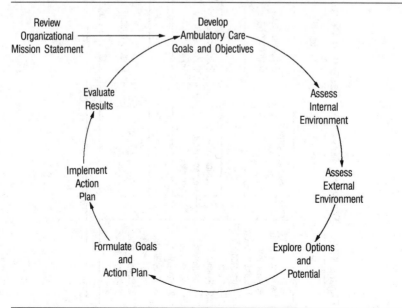

Figure 17-2. Planning Model for Taubman Center Project, University of Michigan Medical Center

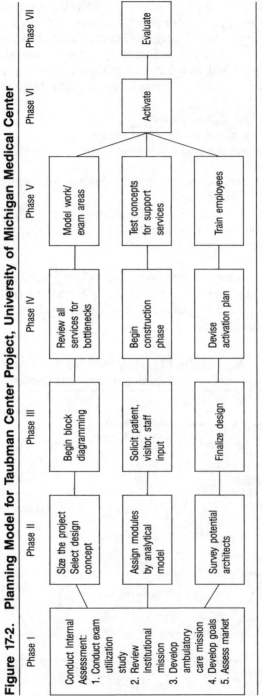

Planning and Evaluating Facility Design

After the mission statement and goals were determined, the next step was to plan and evaluate design considerations.

Planning the Design

Input from patients was a key element in planning the design. A study conducted by the Office of Planning, Research and Development polled patients via focus groups to ask what they liked and disliked about the present facilities. This study was honored by the Design Research Recognition Program of the National Endowment for the Arts.[3-5] Parking that was too distant from the site of the visit and difficulty in accessing the facility from area to area were two problems identified by focus groups. Elements were then incorporated into the plan to address these problems. A new parking structure that holds 1,000 cars was designed so that patients can park on the same floor as their physician's office. The front door was designed to allow convenient patient drop-off and is staffed by door attendants similar to those working in the hotel industry. Door attendants can park a car, help patients to visit clinics by wheelchair, or assist with other needs.

The architects also included a dramatic design feature: a three-story atrium with a skylight that serves as a focal point for the building and as a visual orientation for the patients and visitors. The front of the atrium is the parking structure, and to the rear are the waiting rooms for the clinics. Therefore, the atrium assists visitors in finding their way to services.

The group worked diligently to remove any sign of the old "clinic" mentality. The physicians' offices are located behind open, airy waiting rooms. Lamps, plants, and artwork complete the ambience of the physicians' offices. The response from patients has been extremely positive, with the most common comment being that "the Taubman Center looks more like a fine hotel than a hospital."

Patients also wanted the facility to have a friendly environment. An arts program, one of the few in the country, was designed to include monthly gallery shows in the public areas and an art cart from which inpatients can select artwork for their rooms during their hospital stay. A permanent art collection, live performances, and events such as artist demonstrations are scheduled periodically. This program has had a positive response from visitors, patients, and staff.

Selecting and Evaluating the Design

Each department was involved in selecting and evaluating the design for its area. A modular-design concept was chosen to standardize the project and still allow flexibility for each department. Each module consisted of eight examination rooms and either one treatment room of 200 square feet or two treatment rooms of 100 square feet each. The module also contained clean and dirty linen utility rooms; waiting room space; billing, reception, and clerical support space; storage; consultation space; and a staff room of 500 square feet to support educational activities.

Each department chose to arrange the modules in a different manner. Some departments eliminated treatment rooms in favor of more examination rooms. Should the medical center want to add on to the building and rearrange departments, the modular design allows for such expansion without requiring major changes in the facility's design. A couple of methods allowed each department to evaluate the design and create layouts for the placement of furniture and equipment and examine work space. These methods included using block diagramming and model office designs.

Using Block Diagramming or "Gaming"

For block diagramming (gaming), each department was given a mock-up of their allotted space, as well as colored pieces of paper drawn to scale to represent furniture and equipment used by that department. The module could be "gamed" or laid out in any way desired as long as the square-foot assignment was not changed. Any remaining space could be configured to department specifications.

The department teams for gaming consisted of physicians, nurses, and administrators. The use of the colored blocks helped members of the group who had difficulty reading and interpreting blueprints. The space came alive and was easier to understand.

Using Model Office Designs

Another useful planning method was the designing of three model offices containing new modular furniture. Physicians were allowed to vote on the model they preferred. Many of the offices in the new facility were much smaller than offices in the old facility and required a change of furniture.

The planning committee established the model rooms. The chairmen's offices had 200 square feet; section heads had 150 square feet; and medical staff had 100 square feet. The furniture layouts in three rooms of 100 square feet each allowed the medical staff to test room size and facilitated physician support.

Examination rooms also were developed in model formats so that furniture and sink placement could be planned. Mock cardiopulmonary arrests were set up to test the size of the room as well as the placement of the furniture.

Reviewing the Design and Patient Flow

To facilitate the design process, each of the major departments that would occupy space in the facility was invited to a roundtable planning session.

At each table, a group of support personnel—for example, persons from medical records, radiology, pathology, registration, pharmacy, and administration—joined the department chairman, head nurse, medical director, and design office representative. Each roundtable was assigned to take an imaginary patient from the parking structure through registration, to the clinic, through the check-in process, to the examination room, to diagnostic testing, through check-out, and finally back to the parking structure. Each group was to identify any problems encountered by the patient along the way. The meetings were scheduled to last for two hours. Often discussions continued for more than four hours as people cataloged their responses to the process.

From the lists, planners selected those areas that caused difficulties for patients as they were processed through the various departments. Further in-depth study of these areas allowed for system refinements that minimized patient confusion and stress. Areas that were reviewed fell into the following categories:

- Building signs and self-directing (wayfinding) logos
- Entrance/safety/patient services
- Registration
- Appointments
- Medical records
- Tube system
- Materials management
- Pharmacy
- Transportation of patients and supplies
- Communications
- Laboratory
- Radiology

A task force was formed for each problem area. The assignment was to study the area and prepare a report in the following preestablished format:

- Statement of purpose
- Assumptions of volumes, waiting times, and so forth
- Operational statement
  - Existing problems
  - Desired services
  - Quality standards
- Issues to be resolved

Each task force was asked to review completely its problem area and make suggestions for change. These task forces, which included both design and operational people, allowed the design to proceed in concert with the defining of operations. A final report was generated by each group and circulated throughout the organization for final review. Because of this methodology, many hours of postmove logistical problem solving were eliminated, resulting in the development of new systems that were vast improvements over the old systems.

One problem that was solved was the handling of medical records. The record room was to be located in the basement of the new facility. Dumbwaiters were installed to move records from the record room to a record completion unit on each floor. A computerized medical record locator system was developed to streamline the finding of records. The system allowed personnel to deliver 90 percent of the records on time for clinic visits, including records for patients who were added to the schedule the same day.

Conclusion

The facility opened in February 1986. Since that time, patient visits have grown by more than 200,000. Much of this growth is the result of the consumer-oriented design and customer approval of the new facility.

This project illustrates how change can be facilitated by involving all affected parties in the planning process. Although the process was intensive and time-consuming, the yield has been a superior facility that the entire organization is proud of. The intangible feeling of organizational satisfaction generated by this experience has served as the basis for the continued repositioning of facilities and services at UMMC.

References

1. Bachrach, D., and Marszalek-Gaucher, E. A monumental expansion effort. *Medical Group Management* 32:56, May–June 1985.

2. Eady, C., Bames, S., and others. Characteristics of outpatient room utilization. *Journal of Ambulatory Care Management* 6:43–56, May 1983.

3. Carpman, J. R., Grant, M. A., and Simmons, D. A. *Design That Cares: Planning Health Facilities for Patients and Visitors.* Chicago: American Hospital Publishing, 1986.

4. Carpman, J. R., Grant, M. A., and Simmons, D. A. *No More Mazes: Research about Design for Wayfinding in Hospitals.* Ann Arbor, MI: Office of the Replacement Hospital Program, University of Michigan, 1984.

5. Reizenstein, J. E., and Grant, M. A. *From Hospital Research to Hospital Design: The Patient and Visitor Participation Project.* Ann Arbor, MI: Office of Hospital Planning, Research and Development, University of Michigan, 1982.

Annotated Bibliography

Ambulatory Care Overview

Baliga, B. R., and Johnson, B. Analysis of an industry in transition. *Health Care Strategic Management* 4(12):5–14, Dec. 1986.

> The health care industry is undergoing major structural changes. The significance of these changes for individual competitors in the 1990s is not yet clear. This article assesses the implications of the current changes by applying Michael Porter's industry structure and generic strategy frameworks to the health care industry. Present trends are compared to this analysis to highlight areas in which individual hospitals might improve their competitive positioning.

Clement, J. P. Does hospital diversification improve financial outcomes? *Medical Care* 25(10):988–1001, Oct. 1987.

> Service product diversification is a popular recommendation made to hospitals to increase profitability and reduce financial risk as they face a more hostile reimbursement environment. This article presents results from an empirical study of these claims. Using data from all California not-for-profit hospitals, the study finds that diversification, regardless of whether or not it is related to preexisting services, is not associated with either increased profitability or reduced financial risk. However, other variables that do have these effects, such as physicians per staffed bed and return on assets, are identified in the research. The author suggests that future research should evaluate the effect on financial variables of both the size of the investment and the length of time since the initial diversifying investment.

Coddington, D. C., and Moore, K. D. Diversification offers new opportunities for health care. *Healthcare Financial Management* 41(5):65–66, 68–71, May 1987.

Although many new ventures are struggling and profits are being generated slowly, there are many potentially successful opportunities available to the aggressive health care system. In this article, the authors define diversification, emphasizing its major differences with another "change" tool, incremental changes in the product line. The article also gives the reasons why health care organizations diversify into new businesses, as well as tips on how to successfully implement a diversification strategy, how to develop and test new venture screening criteria, how to perform market segmentation analysis in relation to potential new ventures, and how to develop and maintain realistic expectations concerning the new business's performance. The organizational and financial implications of managing the new venture are discussed, as are the associated strategic implications.

Kirchner, M. What your hospital must do to survive. *Medical Economics* 66(5):152, 154–60, 162, 164–66, Mar. 6, 1989.

In today's turbulent health care environment, hospitals are seeking ways to protect their bottom line and spread their financial risks. They are purchasing in bulk and sharing equipment to cut costs, investing for added revenue, strengthening their financial position through capital and cash-flow pools, forming HMOs and PPOs in an effort to pull in patients, and getting much savvier about marketing. But perhaps most important, they are expanding outpatient services and converting quite a few of their closed acute care beds to new uses. This article explores the ways in which hospitals have ventured beyond their inpatient market, including finding new uses for surplus beds, targeting hospital marketing programs to physicians, joining multihospital systems, developing for-profit subsidiaries, and, most important, expanding their ambulatory care product line. The article provides opinions from various experts in the health care field regarding the various options hospitals can pursue to ward off competition and respond effectively to other environmental influences. In addition, it provides a perspective on how the federal government, Blue Cross/Blue Shield, and commercial insurance plans are planning to reimburse hospitals for these new ventures.

Morris, D. E. Health care entrepreneurs seek profit in diversification. *Texas Hospitals* 41(5):19–21, Mar. 1988.

Shrinking margins in core businesses have motivated health care entrepreneurs to seek investments in a diverse selection of related enterprises.

In this way they can return profits to the bottom line. Experience shows that these ventures must be carefully selected for real profitability. This article provides an overview of the nonacute care segment of the health care market and its potential for future growth and investment opportunities. Some of the diversification options reviewed include nursing homes, health maintenance organizations (HMOs), medical malls, diagnostic clinics, and physician practice acquisition. In addition, the author provides a practical list of do's and don'ts for launching any new hospital venture. Hospital executives will profit most by investing in diversification efforts that support their core business first, and then by seeking entrepreneurial managers and giving them the maximum practical autonomy in seeking and gaining results.

Price, C. Implementing innovation in health care through entrepreneurship. *Topics in Health Records Management* 9(4):5–14, June 1989.

Corporate venturing programs offer one approach to implementing the innovation that the changing health care environment demands. This article focuses on the new venture creations in the health care industry. It is based on an in-depth case survey conducted with the most innovative health care providers in the nation, as well as on extensive interviews and research of the literature. The effects of these new ventures on the corporate culture of health care institutions, financing techniques, marketing strategies, and management implications are addressed. The specifics discussed include the importance of innovation in health care, implementing innovation through corporate venturing, the status of corporate venturing in health care, and the results of corporate venturing in health care organizations.

Rylko-Bauer, B. The development and use of freestanding emergency centers: a review of the literature. *Medical Care Review* 45(1):129–63, Spring 1988.

This article examines the literature concerning freestanding emergency centers (FECs) to assess what they are, who uses them, their current role, and, more important, their future role in the changing delivery system. The first section of the article deals with the development of FECs, examining factors that foster their growth, regulatory constraints, and their various organizational forms. The second section examines patient care and utilization, analyzing user profiles, medical problems treated in FECs, access, quality of care, and cost. The third section examines how FECs fit into the larger health care system, from the standpoint of both integration and competition with other health care providers. The final section discusses how changes in the health care industry will affect FECs. Issues such as diversification, the development of alternative delivery systems and their effects on FECs, and vertical and horizontal integration are discussed.

Sabatino, F. G. The diversification success story continues: survey. *Hospitals* 63(1): 26–32, Jan. 5, 1989.

In 1987, *Hospitals* magazine initiated a survey to examine the profitability of diversification efforts at U.S. hospitals. The results of the survey were published in 1988. This article details the results of a second survey conducted in 1988 by Hamilton/KSA of Atlanta to follow up on the 1987 diversification survey. The latest survey indicates that hospital diversification efforts continue to be successful. Once again, the article provides information on select diversification options on these scales: profit making, a break-even venture, and likelihood of unprofitability. The success of various diversification options is also broken down by geographic region. Other findings include the following: (1) In terms of strategy, an increase in market share—rather than a drive for profitability—is the primary goal of CEOs in establishing priority programs; (2) Priority programs, or designated "centers of excellence," have become a common strategy for hospital CEOs; (3) The effect of competition is more pronounced in the areas of substance abuse treatment and satellite urgent care; (4) More individual medical, women's medicine, and psychiatric treatment programs are experiencing greater financial success than they have in the past; and (5) Sure-fire strategies of the past, such as ambulatory surgery, are making less of a profit.

Sabatino, F. G., and Grayson, M. A. Diversification: more black ink than red ink. *Hospitals* 62(1):36–42, Jan. 5, 1988.

This article summarizes the results of a survey sent to hospital CEOs to determine the profitability and success of 18 various diversification ventures. Out of 2,000 surveys mailed, 353 CEOs responded. The article provides information on these diversification options on three scales: profit making, break-even, and money losing. In addition, these three scales as they relate to all 18 ventures discussed in the article are broken out by region. Finally, the CEOs' preferences for future product line initiatives are discussed.

Snook, I. D. Change brings opportunities for hospital entrepreneurs. *Topics in Hospital Pharmacy Management* 6(4):1–11, Feb. 1987.

The opportunities for change in the hospital industry are far-reaching. These changes are being encouraged by a variety of factors, chiefly the growth in noninvasive technology, competition, changing payment systems, and a greater emphasis on providing cost-effective patient care. Consequently, these changes have created a burgeoning ambulatory care market as hospitals shift from the inpatient to the outpatient side of the patient care equation to protect market share and increase revenues. This article discusses the impacts these changes have had on the health care industry, specifically examining hospitals' responses in the area of new product development. New products examined in the article are hotel-hospitals, comprehensive outpatient rehabilitation facilities (CORFs), home health services, mental health care services, and health care services designed especially for business and industry. In addition, the article details the restructuring of health provider institutions and the hospital of the future.

Facility Design/Planning

Beale, C. Medical mall conveys a 21st century image with room to expand. *Health Facilities Management* 1(1):16–17, Sept. 1988.

This article previews the All Saints-Cityview Medical Mall located in Fort Worth, Texas. The mall is owned by All Saints Healthcare Corporation and its flagship hospital, All Saints Episcopal Hospital. The article discusses the intentions behind constructing the mall, design construction objectives, site selection, the various treatment facilities contained in the mall, the actual design and configuration of the mall, and objectives for future expansion.

Cherskov, M. Hospital design follows the crowd to ambulatory care. *Hospitals* 61(4):58–62, Feb. 20, 1987.

The trend toward ambulatory care is staggering. About $7 billion was spent on hospital construction from September 1985 to September 1986, according to the U.S. Department of Commerce. Of that, $2.5 billion funded ambulatory care projects. In part to accommodate that move toward a consumer-driven health care market, architectural designs are created to appeal to consumers. This article brings together a host of experts and their opinions on the future of hospital design and construction as it relates to ambulatory care. In addition, it addresses the role physicians play in hospital construction and the various approaches used in financing the new facilities. The article cautions that when planning any kind of redesign and construction, hospital planners often make two fundamental mistakes: they look beyond traditional hospital capital resources, and they wait too long before beginning their search.

Craw, J. B. Environmental impact — design with care. *College Review* 6(1):27–44, Spring 1989.

Attention to every detail of the environmental design of the medical group is of extreme importance. Management's familiarity with practice surroundings and layout is often a barrier to scrutinizing it objectively from a patient's point of view. This article presents the results of a study conducted to gather information regarding various aspects of health care facilities, their design, and their environment. A survey was conducted of patients in both rural and urban areas, as was an environmental audit of facilities in both areas. The environmental audit provides a self-assessment tool with which the environmental impact of the practice, regardless of size, can be objectively assessed and critiqued by management. The audit provides a practice with the basis for examining and improving the physical structure and ambience, both internally and externally. The environmental audit instructions and questionnaires are provided in the appendix to the article.

Eubanics, P. Wayfinding: more than just putting up signs. *Health Facilities Management* 2(6):20, 22–23, 25, June 1989.

A new approach to the problem of leading people through any type of building is developing, and its applications to health facilities are just emerging. It is called wayfinding, and it uses an integrated system of visual and architectural cues to help people figure out where they are and where they are going. With wayfinding, such elements as lighting, color, texture, and architecture work together, making the first-time building user feel comfortable in determining how to get from point A to point B. This article discusses the wayfinding concept as it applies to health care facilities, specifically asking facility planners' opinions on the use of wayfinding.

Hansen, R. F. Increasing market share through good design. *Health Care Strategic Management* 4(3):16–21, Mar. 1987.

As they adjust to the pressures of competition, health care executives and trustees are looking for creative ways to position their facilities for future success by using architecture as a marketing tool. The corporate world has for some time used architectural design to achieve marketing goals. This approach is now being used in health care. The author cites examples of hospitals that have used architecture to reach target customers, successfully support efforts at niche marketing, and convey a specific image or message.

Jones, W. J. Letting technology dictate design. *Health Care Strategic Management* 6(11):10–12, Nov. 1988.

Hospitals have two basic choices when embarking on major expansion or renovation projects: they can either let the design of the new structure dictate how the hospital will use the technology it houses or let the technology guide design strategy. This article makes a case for the second option—letting technology dictate design. Specifically, the article provides information on space design for such new technologies as implantable computers, artificial body parts, new testing breakthroughs, and computing as the basis for new diagnostic technologies, to name a few. It also discusses the "program floors" concept, or distinct designated units serving similar patients and "group treatment rooms" for chronic care patients. Overall, managers will need to push for design that will enhance, rather than hinder, existing and future technology.

Remen, S. Master planning: the integration of facilities planning with long-range clinical and financial objectives. *Topics in Health Care Financing* 11(4):57–64, Summer 1985.

Because of the turbulent nature of the health care environment, in which expanded services and new technology are the name of the game, health care professionals must work closely together to accomplish what are essentially interdisciplinary tasks, of which facilities planning represents a significant portion. The article suggests that producing a first-rate master plan that is capable of meeting the stated clinical, financial, and facilities objectives requires a cross-discipline planning team. Components of the master plan include clinical services planning, business and financial planning, and facilities planning. The facilities plan typically includes a survey and analysis of existing conditions, a site survey, a functional analysis, a building systems analysis, strategy development, space programming, and design and block planning. The master plan in general, and the facilities plan in particular, will address issues for the scrutiny of others, and for the guidance of the institution's present and future leaders.

Rostenberg, B. Alternate health care facilities: design reflects quality image. *Trustee* 40(4):15–19, Apr. 1987.

To maintain high-quality services under increasing economic pressure, hospitals are turning to alternate health care delivery facilities, with their lower overhead costs. The challenge for planners is twofold: to attract patients and to provide affordable services without sacrificing quality of care. This article discusses the benefits of creative architectural packaging as it relates to the changing patterns in health care delivery. It emphasizes the importance of visibility, accessibility, image, flexibility, and economy in designing an effective architectural package. The article also discusses how cost containment and new technologies are fueling the growth of nontraditional health care settings.

Financing/Reimbursement

Alternative financing sources. *Health Technology* 1(5):206–11, Sept.–Oct. 1987.

This article describes a variety of capital sources that health care organizations can tap when contemplating the development of a new ambulatory care project, especially high-tech freestanding centers. The structure, advantages, and disadvantages of real estate investment trusts (REITs), master limited partnerships (MLPs), per-use "rentals," and venture capital are discussed. In addition, a discussion of banks as creative capital sources is provided.

Jacobs, P. Financial management in ambulatory care: which costs? *Journal of Ambulatory Care Management* 11(4):88–92, Nov. 1988.

Since the introduction of DRGs, which created cost-cutting incentives for inpatient care, the issue of product-costing for inpatient care has become very popular. In addition, the growth of capitation-type reimbursement and the future implementation of a prospective payment system for outpatient services has created cost-cutting incentives in the ambulatory care market. This article reviews the various purposes for which costing information is necessary, discusses various cost concepts, and shows in a simple example how each is calculated.

Kerschner, M. I., and Rooney, J. M. Utilizing cost accounting information for budgeting. *Topics in Health Care Financing* 13(4):56–66, Summer 1987.

The prospective payment system, the proliferation of alternative delivery systems, and other efforts by third-party payers to reduce acute care utilization have made controlling costs an issue of primary importance for financial managers. This situation has, in turn, led to an increased emphasis on budgeting. This article examines various approaches to the hospital budgeting process, such as traditional budgeting, flexible budgeting, case mix budgeting, and case mix budgeting using cost accounting information.

Lion, J., Malbon, A., and Bergman, A. Ambulatory visit groups: implications for hospital outpatient departments. *Journal of Ambulatory Care Management* 10(1):56–69, Feb. 1987.

As the number of outpatient visits made to hospitals continues to increase, a clinically meaningful classification system that can distinguish among types of patients based on resource consumption is needed to effectively manage and finance hospital outpatient departments. This article focuses on a second-generation derivative of ambulatory patient groups known as ambulatory visit groups (AVGs). The AVGs consist of 571 groups, encompassing ambulatory surgery and tertiary high-technology specialties as well as primary care. A description and evaluation of the system is provided to help health care decision makers to more fully understand the nature of AVGs.

Ring, W. H., and Rufener, B. L. Management of the freestanding surgicenter and the allocation of costs. *Journal of Ambulatory Care Management* 10(1):22–35, Feb. 1987.

One of the most important management tools in a surgicenter is an accurate, useful accounting system that appropriately allocates the cost of running the facility. Without the information that can be generated by such a system, managers may be making decisions without any basis in fact and may be pursuing courses of action that do not benefit the surgicenter. This article reviews the uses of accounting systems and describes a method of allocating costs that can help improve or maintain the profitability of the surgicenter.

Robinson, M. L. Less money, more players in outpatient market. *Hospitals* 63(2):26, 28, 30, Jan. 20, 1989.

Declining reimbursement and increasing competition are making outpatient services less profitable. However, experts contend that with tight cost control, hospitals can still be successful in the outpatient market. This article explores the effects a reduction in reimbursement for outpatient care can have on the delivery of such services. It examines the federal government's initiatives to cut outpatient costs for Medicare beneficiaries and its efforts to implement outpatient prospective payment by 1991. In addition, it discusses the notion of pricing at the margin to service cutbacks in payment and the effect that competition from freestanding clinics has on hospital-based facilities. Finally, it illustrates how various hospitals are developing tactical solutions to the cutbacks in outpatient reimbursement.

Information Systems

Batchelor, G. J., Butler, P. W., and Jellinek, L. A. Clinical profiles manage quality, cost of hospital product. *Healthcare Financial Management* 41(7):66–69, 72, July 1987.

This article explores the bottom line of patient classification systems—their ability to measure the consumption and the quality of health care services. The authors have used physician-specified clinical profiles as a method of measurement. These profiles delineate the appropriate number and mix of services needed to deliver care to specific groups of patients, the structural elements that provide efficient and effective delivery of care, and the expected outcome measure for evaluating care. The results of a study conducted by the authors at Rush-Presbyterian-St. Luke's Medical Center in Chicago to develop physician-specified clinical profiles are discussed. The article provides information on the profile development process and on the applications of these profiles for product definition and pricing, utilization management, describing and monitoring quality, marketing, program planning and budgeting, and as a teaching tool.

Borgess turnaround more dramatic than previously told. *National Report on Computers and Health* 10(10):4–5, May 15, 1989.

Borgess Medical Center (Kalamazoo, MI) has increased its market share from 15.5 percent to 21.2 percent and expanded its service area from 9 to 16 counties using physician networking. According to the president of Michigan Healthcare Network, a Borgess subsidiary, the 462-bed hospital has had a net return on investment of $3.4 million in 1987 and $2.4 million in 1986. Of 400 physicians on staff, 130 are directly involved in the network, with an additional 165 physicians referring patients to the 130. The hospital provides computers and software to the physicians at no charge. Services available include laboratory and radiology findings, accounts receivable, insurance billing, and practice-management software.

Cohn, D. M., and Shaw, P. L. Development of outpatient data bases. *Computers in Healthcare* 9(4):88–89, Apr. 1988.

The implementation of a prospective payment system (PPS) for outpatients will have a significant impact on hospital operations and the development of information systems. This article discusses the reimbursement environment that will take effect under an outpatient prospective payment system as it relates to management information needs. It provides information on designing and implementing a strategy to develop an outpatient data base. Specifically, it gives guidelines on building and maintaining the data base, determining data needs, and reviewing the completeness, timeliness, and data quality of the outpatient medical record.

Donovan, W. PCs in group practice. *Group Practice Journal* 38(3):8–9, 12–14, 16–17, May–June 1989.

The three areas of immediate interest to the group practice are knowledge retrieval, division support, and continuing education capabilities to aid the practicing physician. A fourth one that is becoming even more important is the networking of physicians' computers with other health information systems. This article explores the present and future use of personal computers (PCs) in the group practice setting, examining such new applications as telephone-linked computer (TLC) systems, cellular services, satellite images, artificial intelligence, medical computing, and paperless submission of claims. In addition, the article provides case studies of the applications in use and researches ventures into new areas of computer applications.

Gans, D. W. Medical group information systems. *Medical Group Management Journal* 37(2):11, 55–56, 58, Mar.–Apr. 1989.

This article reports and summarizes the results of a survey of information resource management in medical group practices sponsored by the Center for Research in Ambulatory Health Care Administration and the Healthcare Specialized Practice Unit of Price Waterhouse. The article provides information on the relative market penetration of manufacturers, major criteria considered in the selection process, most commonly used applications, and future computer applications.

Hospital-physician bonding: the computer connection. *Health Technology* 2(5):189–95, Sept.–Oct. 1988.

Hospitals seeking ways to increase their utilization must not overlook the medical staff, who form the main channel for patient admissions and referrals. Because physicians generally admit patients where they feel the best care is offered — and where their practice of medicine is most facilitated — many hospitals wishing to attract and retain physicians have linked patient data to physicians' offices via computer. This article explains how physicians' offices can be linked with hospital information systems, the economic justifications for linking hospitals and physicians via an information system, and the legal issues and risks surrounding the decision.

Malhortra, N. K. Decision support systems for health care marketing managers. *Journal of Health Care Marketing* 9(2):20–28, June 1989.

Health care organizations are encouraged to implement decision support systems geared to meeting the challenges of tomorrow. This article outlines a decision support system (DSS) and illustrates its usefulness for health care marketing managers. A schematic representation of DSS is described. Applications of DSS in strategic marketing and planning, product, promotion, and distribution decisions are discussed. Potential problems of integrating DSS into health care organizations are identified and some useful guidelines for implementation are offered.

Packer, C. L. Integration, performance key to ambulatory care information systems. *Hospitals* 59(10):120–22, May 16, 1985.

The integration of patient registration and scheduling, billing and accounts receivable, procedure coding, physician billing, and results reporting is crucial for ambulatory care information management. This article examines several ambulatory care data-processing functions and reports on hospital experiences with these functions. The results are compared to previously reported data for more traditional hospital data-processing activities. The article illustrates the differences between the traditional activities in data processing and those designed to support ambulatory care.

Pearce, D. Decision support. Key executives speak out. *Computers in Health-care* 8(8):26–35, Aug. 1987.

The author interviewed 12 executives from various hospitals across the country on their data needs. Those interviewed discussed the obvious need for more sophisticated and technologically advanced decision support systems. The interviewees also identified the need to model future management information systems to coincide with their visions of the future health care system model, to share information between physician practices and their organizations, and to provide shared data bases of noncompetitive information among health care providers and between providers and insurance carriers to ease the costs and financial risks of admissions, billing, insurance verification, and scheduling.

Roth, M. Computer contracting for ambulatory care providers. *Journal of Ambulatory Care Management* 12(2):67–74, May 1989.

Ambulatory care providers increasingly will rely on sophisticated computer systems to perform many, if not most, financial and patient care record-keeping functions and related analyses that previously were performed manually. Computers also will be used increasingly by ambulatory care providers to conduct systemwide utilization reviews. Given these and other essential functions that computers will perform, ambulatory care providers will need to pay serious heed to the phrase *caveat emptor* ("let the buyer beware") when they contract to purchase computer systems. In order to protect an ambulatory care provider's long-term interests, the contract to purchase a computer system must include essential protections that are not routinely incorporated in the computer vendor's standard contract. This article discusses elements that should be included in a contract in order to safeguard the financial interests of the ambulatory care provider that purchases a computer system. Items discussed include licensure, source code, installation schedule, suitability of premises, warranty, maintenance and repairs, and purchase price.

Somand, M. The computerized medical record in a multisite ambulatory setting. *Topics in Health Records Management* 8(3):17–22, Mar. 1988.

The growth of offsite ambulatory care facilities poses a particular problem regarding the flow of medical information. Issues of access, transportation, and timing all make management of medical records more complex than it was in the single-site institution. This article discusses the actions taken by the Henry Ford Health Care Corporation to integrate the flow of medical information across its inpatient facilities, outpatient facilities, and its other affiliated organizations. Specifically, it provides information on the Computer Stored Ambulatory Record (COSTAR) System. The article puts into perspective the operational aspects of the COSTAR system, the methodology used to evaluate the effectiveness of the system, and the perceived future role of the COSTAR system in the Henry Ford Health Care Corporation's operating environment.

Steinwachs, D. M. Ambulatory care management information systems: future directions. *Journal of Ambulatory Care Management* 8(2):84–94, May 1985.

As payment systems change and competitive pressures begin to mount, ambulatory care facilities require information that can guide efforts to enhance provider productivity, enlarge market share, and improve the overall efficiency and effectiveness of the facility. This article focuses on the methodological issues in the application of management information systems to these new and emerging management concerns.

Toole, J. E., and Caine, M. E. Laying a foundation for future information systems. *Topics in Health Care Financing* 14(2):17–27, Winter 1987.

As the health care industry continues to restructure itself, health care facilities are simultaneously restructuring their management information systems. Hospital data processing can no longer get by merely with paying employees, keeping the books, and processing routine financial data. This article describes a process hospitals can use when redesigning their information systems. It provides information on developing a plan of action, identifying institutional direction and requirements, choosing the right hardware/software strategy, assessing future technology, choosing a vendor, and developing a transition plan.

Joint Ventures

Brice, J. Pulling together. Hospitals, doctors team up to fight financial, legal odds. *HealthWeek* 2(9):17–21, Apr. 25, 1988.

Joint ventures between hospitals and physicians are a volatile, controversial, and increasingly common way of pursuing business opportunities in health care. Analysts say that hundreds of such ventures, with varying missions, configurations, and potential for success, are formed each year. But despite their obvious and growing popularity, not all joint ventures enjoy smooth sailing. There is the risk of failure, legal ramifications, and ethical concerns. The article provides a brief overview of the joint venture business, focusing on such issues as fitting joint ventures into a hospital's strategic plan, partnership formation patterns, state regulation of hospital–physician joint ventures, types of joint ventures, and the avoidance of legal problems, to name a few.

Cowart, R. G., and Freeman, K. M. Mobile, high-technology joint ventures. *Journal of Ambulatory Care Management* 11(4):15–22, Nov. 1988.

Many community hospitals and ambulatory care centers cannot afford individually to own and operate expensive high-technology equipment. Consequently, they are turning to a variety of medical care providers to joint venture such equipment on a mobile basis as a means of guaranteeing utilization and spreading financial risk. This article discusses the cooperative means for achieving a fair arrangement among institutions interested in joint venturing in mobile, high-technology equipment. It provides information on such topics as technology selection, medical staff participation, site issues, scheduling, payment considerations, and regulatory issues.

DeMuro, P. R. Joint ventures for mobile equipment reduce hospital costs. *Healthcare Financial Management* 43(4):52, 56, 58, 60, 62, 64, Apr. 1989.

Many hospitals cannot afford to purchase all of the high-technology equipment necessary to provide a full range of services. Health care organizations should consider entering into a joint venture to gain access to mobile equipment. However, changes pending in Washington dictate caution for all health care joint ventures, particularly those involving physician investments. This article reviews and discusses such issues as selecting participants, operational issues, legal issues, and the development of a joint venture checklist.

Harpster, L. M. Planning an ambulatory care joint venture. *The Medical Staff Counselor* 2(3):49–55, Summer 1988.

This article discusses ambulatory care joint ventures by hospitals and selected members of their medical staff and emphasizes the resolution of problems in the early planning stages. The author emphasizes that failure to follow an orderly and thoughtful planning process not only risks valuable resources of the venture partners, but also jeopardizes the working relationship between the hospital and its medical staff. In addition, the article discusses the issue of control of the business once it becomes operational.

Joseph, J. M. Hospital joint ventures: charting a safe course through a sea of antitrust regulations. *American Journal of Law and Medicine* 13(4):621–24, 1989.

Recent changes in the health care industry, including rapidly rising costs, increased competition, and new methods of reimbursement, have forced hospitals to create new strategies for remaining competitive. One of the more recent innovations is the joint venture. Although joint ventures can greatly enhance a hospital's competitive edge, if courts find that joint ventures produce illegal price fixing, illegal boycotts, or monopolistic activities, this competitive innovation may be prohibited under the Sherman or Clayton Acts. This article focuses on potential antitrust conflicts that could arise during hospital participation in joint ventures. Various precautions that may ensure the legality of a hospital's joint venture are suggested. The article also examines joint ventures between hospitals, or between a hospital and a group of physicians, that sell a product or provide a service. This article also summarizes methods of analyzing entities under applicable antitrust laws.

Rublee, D. A. Joint ventures in medical services. *The Journal of Medical Practice Management* 2(3):154–60, Winter 1987.

This article is an overview of joint venture activity in health care, describing trends in joint ventures and raising issues for physicians. The article discusses the major facets of joint venture alliances and identifies policy issues that arise from the trend to use joint ventures as an organizational tool. In addition, speculation is made about the future role of joint ventures in the organization of health care.

Zasa, R. J., and Unger, J. L. Planning joint ventures of ambulatory surgical centers and primary care centers: avoiding the pitfalls. *Journal of Ambulatory Care Management* 11(4):28–32, Nov. 1988.

This article outlines the activities recommended during the predevelopment phase of strategic joint venturing of ambulatory surgical and primary care centers. It discusses the role of market feasibility studies, financial feasibility reports, development groups or teams, and the selection of partners. It also provides information on the ownership and organization of the joint venture, as well as on methods of financing the venture.

Zisner, D., McCally, J. F., Zagaria, J. D., and others. Successful joint ventures for today's competitive health care marketplace. *Group Practice Journal* 37(5):27, 30, 35, 38, 40, Sept.–Oct. 1988.

Hospitals and physicians alike have come to the conclusion that mutual economic and financial cooperation is essential if they are to survive and prosper in this highly competitive health care marketplace. This article discusses the basis for successful hospital–physician joint ventures. It provides information on strategic market objectives, guiding principles for an effective physician–hospital joint venture, legal issues, reimbursement considerations, and tax considerations. It also gives data on what motivates partners to form a joint venture, the most popular types of joint ventures, and the distribution of types of joint venture partners.

Legal Issues

Beautyman, M. A primer on the reorganization of health care facilities. *Health Care Strategic Management* 5(12):19–20, Dec. 1987.

A reorganization involves the creation of one or more entities that are separate and distinct from the health care facility, each of which performs a specified function. Reorganization may involve either the creation of a parent holding company or the creation of new subsidiaries of a health care facility or new freestanding entities. The article highlights some of the reasons why health care facilities undergo reorganization, specifically examining benefits associated with third-party reimbursement, protection of assets, minimization of regulatory control, increased access to capital, and increased management efficiency. All of these benefits are discussed as they relate to the legal ramifications of corporate restructuring.

Burda, D. Recruitment schemes risk tax status, break law. *Hospitals* 61(11): 48–49, June 5, 1987.

Some popular physician recruitment strategies can result in not-for-profit hospitals losing their federal tax exemption or breaking state laws. As hospitals rush into the marketplace to attract high-admitting physicians, they must alert themselves to the legal ramifications of such activities. This article provides an overview of legal guidelines that the hospital should adhere to in its recruiting practices. Chief among these are guidelines for physician payment, group practice acquisition, and the use of trust funds in buying practices.

Cohen, I., and Kaufman, K. D. Safe harbors from Medicare fraud and abuse sanctions. *Journal of Ambulatory Care Management* 12(2): 1–9, May 1989.

Physicians are becoming increasingly concerned about the applicability of the Medicare antifraud and abuse rules to many of their business arrangements. Recognizing the need for members of the health care industry to be confident about the legality of many of their commercial arrangements under the fraud and abuse rules, Congress included a provision in the Medicare and Medicaid Patient and Program Protection Act of 1987 that requires the secretary of the Department of Health and Human Services to ensure safe harbor regulations specifying which payment practices will not be treated as violations of the Medicare antifraud and abuse rules. This article examines the effect of these safe harbors on ambulatory care joint ventures. First, it summarizes existing federal Medicare antifraud and abuse rules and the recently proposed safe harbor regulations. Next, the article examines the effect of several of the proposed safe harbor provisions on ambulatory care joint ventures. Finally, the article discusses the application of the proposed safe harbor regulations in planning for joint ventures with providers or suppliers.

Cornwell, D. Tax planning for unrelated business income. *Topics in Health Care Financing* 14(4):15–21, Summer 1988.

As hospitals venture outside the acute or inpatient care side of the health care equation, they will continue to rub up against the legal problems associated with unrelated business income (UBI). This is especially the case in nonpatient service areas (such as personnel or data processing).

This article provides information on UBI that tax-exempt health care organizations should recognize and act on. It provides a basic definition of UBI, discusses the sale of nonpatient services to other institutions, defines the rules governing debt-financed income and property, and illustrates how to compute and report UBI.

Goldsmith, S. B. Ambulatory care: emerging legal issues. *The Medical Staff Counselor* 2(1):41–45, Winter 1988.

Several recent cases illustrate how changes in the world of ambulatory health care can lead providers, insurers, organizations, and patients into costly and time-consuming legal maneuvers. This article reviews recent developments in ambulatory care that form the backdrop to these legal cases.

Heller, D. L. Structuring ambulatory care projects to minimize problems with regulatory constraints. *Journal of Ambulatory Care Management* 11(4):23–27, Nov. 1988.

In planning an ambulatory care project, it is very important to structure it so as to minimize problems with the various applicable state and federal regulatory constraints. Failure to do so in advance, using experienced consultants and legal counsel, often results in severe problems and expenses that could have been avoided. This article discusses a variety of regulatory constraints affecting ambulatory care projects, including certificate of need/licensing, illegal remuneration, reimbursement, and securities laws.

Paulson, W. A. Antitrust exposure from joint venture activities. *Journal of Ambulatory Care Management* 11(4):33–43, Nov. 1988.

As health care markets become increasingly competitive, and as physicians and hospitals attempt to consolidate market shares or protect against new entrants in the market, more and more private antitrust suits will be filed. This is especially the case with joint venture arrangements. However, as with any risk, the risks involved in potential antitrust liability can be minimized. If they are not considered in planning, antitrust liabilities can sound the death knell for a business venture. This article examines federal and state antitrust laws as they relate to the creation and implementation of joint ventures. It discusses general antitrust considerations, exclusive dealing arrangements, pricing products and services, market identification and allocation, and noncompetition agreements.

Robey, P. E., and Valiant, C. Safe harbor regulations. Stuck on a shoal. *Group Practice Journal* 38(3):34–38, May–June 1989.

In January of 1989, the Office of the Inspector General (OIG) of the Department of Health and Human Services (HHS) issued proposed regulations defining safe payment practices that are not subject to criminal prosecution under the Medicare and Medicaid antikickback law. These regulations were mandated by the Medicare and Medicaid Patient and Program Protection Act of 1987, which required HHS to promulgate regulations specifying permissible payment practices, or "safe harbors," which are not violative of the antikickback law even though they are potentially capable of inducing referrals of Medicare business. This article provides a perspective on these proposed regulations. It analyzes the language of the antikickback law; interprets the proposed ruling; discusses such safe harbor provisions as space and equipment rental, sale of professional practices, and personal services and management contracts; and analyzes those practices that may fall outside the rule.

Marketing

Van Doren, D. C., and Spielman, A. P. Hospital marketing: strategy reassessment in a declining market. *Journal of Health Care Marketing* 9(1):15–24, Mar. 1989.

Despite continued significant increases in the nation's spending for health care, use of inpatient hospital services has declined. The authors use the product life cycle to analyze the market for hospital services and to examine competitive strategies for hospital marketing success. The article describes in detail four strategies to use for products in decline: exploit growth segments, improve product quality and innovate, improve efficiency, and harvest. The authors analyze the advantages and disadvantages of these strategies as they relate to the hospital market.

Zipin, M. L. Developing a strategic marketing plan. *Health Care Strategic Management* 7(6):13–15, June 1989.

Any strategic planning effort requires careful planning and a systematic approach, and strategic planning is essential to the survival of today's hospital. Whether the hospital is an academic medical center, a community hospital, or some other type of organization, the key to success is a thorough market-planning process. This article describes a four-phase process hospitals can use in preparing a strategic marketing plan.

Phase 1 is the development of a marketing data base and secondary market research, phase 2 is primary market research, phase 3 is the formulation of goals and strategies, and phase 4 is the development of a marketing action plan. The article provides an in-depth discussion of each of these phases.

Marketing Ambulatory Care

Bradshaw, T. M., and Zobin, A. Documentation of effective marketing for a same-day surgery center. *Journal of Health Care Marketing* 7(2):65–69, June 1987.

In an effort to increase the utilization of their same-day surgery program, LaCrosse Lutheran Hospital in LaCrosse, Wisconsin, developed a study to determine physician satisfaction and awareness levels associated with the same-day surgery unit. The target population was all Gunderson Clinic physicians, a group practice adjoining the hospital. The questionnaire was designed to elicit information from the physicians relating to convenience in using the unit, patient satisfaction with care, the strengths and weaknesses of the unit, and receipt of adequate and appropriate information about the unit. The responses received were used by the hospital to modify its scheduling procedures, add an additional preoperative and postoperative care room, and implement an informational campaign to increase the community's awareness of the unit.

McCue, P. Marketing considerations for diagnostic imaging centers. *Medicenter Management* 5(2):20–23, Feb. 1988.

Diagnostic imaging centers face competition from a variety of health care facilities as they vie for position in the marketplace. In this article, several radiologists and business managers involved in existing or planned centers discuss their marketing strategies, modality choices, organizational structure, and other issues pertinent to the operation of a viable freestanding center.

Maurer, M. P. Marketing planning for ambulatory care: twelve key steps. *Journal of Ambulatory Care Marketing* 1(1):3–11, Spring–Summer 1987.

A marketing plan lays out the specific steps for marketing the service in question. This article outlines 12 key steps for developing and writing marketing plans for ambulatory care. The steps discussed include identifying the marketing mission, developing marketing goals/objectives, conducting a marketing audit, evaluating opportunities and threats, market segmentation, market targeting, market positioning, designing appropriate marketing strategies/targets, financial analysis, creating a performance time line, identifying the responsible marketing administration, and providing or developing a control system.

Murphy, R. F. Venture profile analysis. *Hospital and Health Services Administration* 30(6):80–95, Nov.–Dec. 1985.

The venture profile analysis is presented as a low-cost, orderly process to help hospital chief executive officers and governing boards plan for service diversification. Potential business ventures are assigned a weighted score based on nine evaluation criteria (reimbursement, market size, capital costs, competitors, staffing, image, positive spin-offs, certificate of need, and compatibility with the hospital's role). These criteria are then used to assign a weighted score that is used to gauge the prospects of success for the ventures under consideration. The author indicates that the process is intended only as a preliminary screening tool for ranking ventures in relation to predetermined benchmarks and a hospital's limited supply of capital. The article provides examples of how the venture profile analysis can be used to ensure successful market-based planning.

Rosenstein, A. Cost-effective analysis in selection of hospital alternative programs. *Journal of Hospital Marketing* 1(3/4):51–60, Spring–Summer 1987.

The purpose of cost-benefit analysis is to promote cost-effective decision making and optimal allocation of resources in an environment that emphasizes cost containment and reduction of excess capacity. As an economic tool, cost-benefit analysis is designed to provide the administrator with the capability to conduct comparisons between program alternatives on the basis of operational costs versus benefits from revenues gained. As hospitals begin to diversify into new product lines and service areas, an economic analysis of the viability of these diversification ventures is required. This article explores the use of cost-benefit analysis in measuring the quantitative and qualitative impacts of program alternatives.

Rosko, M. D., and Broyles, R. W. Strategic hospital marketing responses to prospective payment. *Journal of Hospital Marketing* 1(3/4):71–81, Spring–Summer 1987.

This article demonstrates how marketing efforts can be used to alter the patient mix of the hospital in order to maximize income or minimize losses. The decision to use marketing to alter patient mix is based on the observation that the major sources of inpatient admissions emanate either from decisions implemented by physicians or from ambulatory service programs of the hospital. The article discusses such issues as using outpatient services to alter patient mix, diffused marketing strategies, marketing mix considerations for outpatient services, physician-related strategies, and the use of alternate delivery systems as a means to alter patient mix.

Scheuerman, J. L., and Fallon, B. Competitive analysis: sizing up the shape of your opponents. *Healthcare Financial Management* 42(9):33–34, 36, 38–40, Sept. 1988.

To survive in an increasingly competitive industry, many health care organizations are struggling to strengthen their performance and position. However, many providers find they lack the internal ability to systematically collect and analyze market and industry information. By using the competitive analysis process described in this article, hospitals can examine current and future market information, which includes insights on industry potential, competition among hospitals with similar characteristics, and the individual hospital's performance. By competitively assessing the industry and themselves, hospitals can position themselves in fresh markets and predict their likely success.

Operational Issues

Berl, R. L., Hooper, R., and Sweeney, R. E. Product lines in a hospital emergency room. *Journal of Ambulatory Care Marketing* 2(2):9–33, 1988.

A hospital's emergency department is not a single product, but is a product system made up of multiple product lines. Although the same department staff deals with all product lines, the return on investment (ROI) for time and resources varies widely among the lines. Each line draws upon a different expertise in the hospital staff and services a different market. Identification of market niches within the broad system of emergency services will enable a hospital to narrow the focus of its marketing efforts to those lines for which a current need can be shown. This article discusses a wide variety of issues relevant to the development of product lines in an emergency department. It examines pricing strategies, product line characteristics, and responses to changing emergency services needs.

Bristol, I., Sepulveda, T., and Lyon, M. Streamlining the preop process. *Health Progress* 70(1):86–87, Jan.–Feb. 1989.

As same-day surgery becomes a mainstay of surgical care, many hospitals are struggling to develop programs to deal with the stress inherent in the rapid admission and discharge of patients. The need to quickly and efficiently perform physical assessments and gather laboratory and diagnostic information, combined with the pressure to prepare patients for surgery soon after admission, puts the hospital, the physician, and the staff under great strain and some risk. The article describes the preoperative program (POP) at Saint John's Hospital and Health Center in Santa Monica, California, which has proved highly successful. The authors provide information on designing the program, implementing the program, and fine-tuning and enhancing the components of the program, as well as an evaluation of the program.

Cole, G., and Brown, C. Product-line management: concept to reality. *Topics in Health Care Financing* 14(3):62–75, Spring 1988.

Product line management, a concept that originated in the manufacturing industry, has been overwhelmingly selected by hospital leaders as a necessary vehicle for becoming more market-driven, improving competitive position, and increasing profitability. This article describes Scripps Memorial Hospital's program line management, an adaptation of the product line concept. The program line management approach is a hybrid of four product line management models that have emerged in the health care industry; the strategic business unit model, the distribution model, the market management model, and the coordinated care model. The program described in the article emphasizes the implementation process within the context of the demands of the local market structure in southern California and the driving forces of the corporate culture at Scripps Memorial Hospital.

Manning, M. F. Product line management: will it work in health care? *Healthcare Financial Management* 41(1):23, 25–29, Jan. 1987.

Although borrowed from the manufacturing sector, product line management can provide a meaningful framework for defining and managing the activities of a health care organization. This article emphasizes the importance of hospitals' developing a productand market-management orientation to keep pace with changes in the health care delivery system and the channels of access to that system. The author states that the development of a meaningful set of product line definitions that accurately reflect the unique characteristics of the hospital's services, markets, and competitive environment is not only the logical first step in this process, but also is critical to the successful transition to a product line approach and future operational viability.

Parrinello, K., Brenner, P. S., and Vallone, B. Refining and testing a nursing patient classification instrument in ambulatory care. *Nursing Administration Quarterly* 13(1):54–65, Fall 1988.

This article provides the findings of a study designed to refine and test a nursing patient classification instrument for ambulatory care at the University of Rochester's Strong Memorial Hospital. The intent behind patient classification instruments is to identify, measure, or classify the nursing needs of patients in ambulatory care settings so as to effectively manage human and fiscal resources associated with patient care. With the explosion in volume and diversity of ambulatory care services provided, it is essential for nurse managers to gain a better understanding of nursing care requirements and the allocation of resources in ambulatory care settings. The article provides information on the conceptual background and purpose of the study, the methodology used, the study findings, and recommendations for further research. Applications of the study findings to clinical practice are also provided.

Patterson, P. OR directors plan strategies for new outpatient PPS. *OR Manager* 3(12):1, 4–5, Dec. 1987.

Operating room directors and hospital financial managers must develop strategies for coping with the transition to a system of Medicare prospective payment for hospital-based outpatient surgery. Although predicting the precise impact of this new reimbursement policy is difficult, many managers are looking for more sophisticated financial information in order to assess their present capacity to handle the transition and model future strategies to accommodate it. This article examines three primary issues that will confront operating room directors and financial managers in this new payment environment. These issues are (1) the decision to organize outpatient surgery services as an integrated or freestanding center; (2) getting a handle on costs and unbundling charges; and (3) reexamining practice patterns in order to successfully compete with freestanding centers. Throughout the article, the comments and opinions of many operating room managers regarding the new payment system are provided.

Rooney, J. New ventures create challenges for the management team. *Healthcare Financial Management* 41(8):46–48, 50–51, Aug. 1987.

The pursuit of opportunities outside traditional inpatient services has resulted in new challenges for the hospital management team. To ensure success, it is important that members of the hospital management team understand their roles in the development and implementation of these new ventures. This article describes the various types of new ventures hospitals are capitalizing on, including those unrelated to health care delivery. In addition, the article discusses the structure of these new venture models, factors critical to their success, and the composition and role of the new venture team. A detailed analysis of the individual participants in the venture team is also provided.

Zasa, R. J. Critical management factors for ambulatory surgery centers. *Medical Group Management Journal* 36(2):28–29, 31, 33, Mar.–Apr. 1989.

Monitoring critical success factors is a management tool that helps managers focus on fundamentals of a particular business. The concept emphasizes delineating the factors that managers believe are critical for that business. It also emphasizes understanding the fundamental factors that will help that business achieve success in areas of quality, personnel, and any other factors that contribute to the success of that business. The article takes the concept of critical success factors and applies it to ambulatory surgery centers. It outlines the data elements that an ambulatory surgery center should capture in order to compare and contrast its performance record. Data elements discussed include man-hours per patient, medical supply expense per patient, number of accounts receivable days uncollected, and operating income, to name a few.

Productivity Assessment

Anderson, T. D. Special issues in productivity programs. *Topics in Health Care Financing* 15(3):31–42, Spring 1989.

Within any hospital there is obviously a large and diverse array of services, functions, and departments requiring both operational and strategic management. Although some crucial issues are shared by virtually all of these areas, there are many distinct characteristics specific to each department within the modern hospital that require individualized knowledge, experience, and actions. This article reviews some of the mutual underlying issues in hospital productivity programs, and then discusses some of the typical issues that must be addressed on a department-by-department basis.

Antle, D. W., and Reid, R. A. Managing service capacity in an ambulatory care clinic. *Hospital and Health Services Administration* 33(2):201–11, Summer 1988.

Capacity management is an essential element of efficient ambulatory care delivery. It seeks to improve organizational effectiveness and productivity by increasing operational efficiency and reducing patient congestion. This article discusses two service capacity management strategies: demand smoothing and supply matching. It also provides the results of a clinic-based study conducted to determine the characteristics of patient flow, including the identification of the major factors responsible for clinic congestion and reviewing the present use of patient examination rooms. Rather than increase the clinical resource base, a balanced set of relevant low-cost strategies is proposed to improve performance.

Boyd, S. D., Coven, B., and Kurth, E. Productivity considerations in the development of a new program and the ongoing management of an outpatient rehabilitation center. *Journal of Ambulatory Care Management* 11(1):34–40, Feb. 1988.

In 1983, Saint Joseph Hospital and Health Care Center in Chicago established and transferred outpatient rehabilitation referrals to the Rehabilitation and Fitness Center, a freestanding outpatient rehabilitation center affiliated with the hospital. The rationale for this was to allow for maximum treatment of inpatients at the hospital and maximum growth of outpatient therapy. This article reviews the development and implementation of the program, focusing on decisions regarding facility design, equipment needs, personnel requirements, and program components. In addition, information is provided on the development and implementation of a productivity system that not only will assist administrators in monitoring and controlling staffing needs, but also will aid them in projecting growth and determining needs for additional staffing and equipment.

DeGuchi, J. J., Inui, T. S., and Martin, D. P. Measuring provider productivity in ambulatory care. *Journal of Ambulatory Care Management* 7(2):29–37, May 1984.

Focusing on patient scheduling systems is one approach used to optimize the use of provider time. This article reports the results of a study conducted by the Seattle Veterans Administration Medical Center to test the comparative impact of centralized and decentralized scheduling on clinic productivity. Information is provided on the setting and background of the study, measures and methods used, the results, and managerial implications. Overall, the study results indicate that the change from a centralized to a decentralized scheduling system was associated with increased productivity of the clinic staff in the aggregate and for each type of specialist.

Hurdle, S., and Pope, G. C. Improving physician productivity. *Journal of Ambulatory Care Management* 12(1):11–26, Feb. 1989.

Today, interest in improving physician productivity is maintained by the high cost of physician services. Using data collected in 1984 and 1985, the authors updated the findings of physician productivity studies conducted during the 1970s. Multivariate analyses of these data showed that many of the key factors previously found to influence physician productivity were still important in the mid-1980s. These variables were group size, employment status of physicians, prepayment to physicians or organizations for medical services, and variations in physician training or skill. The article reviews the impacts of these key physician and practice characteristics on physician productivity. The authors also generate simple descriptive statistics using these same data to highlight differences between productive and unproductive physicians.

Nathanson, S. N. Managing resources effectively in a hospital-based ambulatory surgery program. *Journal of Ambulatory Care Management* 11(1):63–71, Feb. 1988.

Changes in Medicare payment and billing methods for hospital-based ambulatory surgery programs will present challenges to the hospital industry to provide care in the most efficient and cost-effective manner. The article discusses the three parameters of resource management that typically should be considered: labor, equipment and supplies, and facilities. The outcome of efficient management of these resources should be higher quality of care, reduced costs, and increased patient satisfaction.

Reid, R. A., and Antle, D. W. Effective ambulatory service capacity management. *DRG Monitor* 6(5):1–8, Jan. 1989.

An effective capacity management program can increase operational productivities while reducing patient congestion. A framework for ambulatory care capacity management is presented that includes both demand-smoothing and supply-matching strategies. A case study focuses on analyzing congestion in the patient care delivery process at a medical oncology outpatient clinic. Through the use of a balanced and coordinated set of capacity management strategies, a low-cost approach to improved performance may be designed.

Rudnick, J. D. A process and considerations for activating a quality/productivity monitoring system. *Health Care Strategic Management* 5(3): 23–27, Mar. 1987.

In response to demands for cost containment in operational areas without subsequent declines in quality, many hospitals are implementing quality and productivity monitoring systems. This article describes the process used by one hospital to determine that it would use an outside consultant to implement a productivity/monitoring system. This article offers practical advice for other hospitals considering using outside services for developing quality/productivity monitoring systems as well as other projects.

Ventrone, J. M., Zanotti, M., and Heidtman, M. Dressing for success: measuring productivity can ensure continuing success. *Healthcare Financial Management* 42(8):30–32, 34, 36–38, 40, Aug. 1988.

Both managerial and financial benefits can be gained by implementing and monitoring productivity standards in health care organizations. This article discusses one hospital's decision to develop a productivity measuring system. It provides information on the benefits of productivity analyses and the options available in developing productivity standards, specifically focusing on the use of logging or staff recording of time spent on each task performed. The article concludes by discussing the use of the logging process as a tool to manage operational productivity.

Prospective Payment Initiatives

Gildea, J. Toil and trouble over outpatient prospective payment. *Health Cost Management* 5(1):1–10, Jan.–Feb. 1988.

By April 1, 1991, a prospective payment system (PPS) model for reimbursing all Medicare outpatient services is to be ready for implementation. Patient classification systems, which are an integral component of any PPS methodology, are being designed to predict ambulatory resource use (and thus patient costs), but the first to be applied in an actual payment system has just begun demonstrations. This article provides information on the various methods presently available to decision makers who are considering the implementation of an outpatient PPS. The article specifically discusses the promises and pitfalls behind ambulatory visit groups (AVGs), products of ambulatory care (PAC), and emergency department groups (EDGs). In addition, it gives the thoughts of third-party payers regarding these systems and the progress they have made in implementing outpatient prospective payment systems.

Gold, M. Common sense on extending DRG concepts to pay for ambulatory care. *Inquiry* 25(2):281–89, Summer 1988.

The development of Medicare's prospective payment system has led to considerable interest in expanding case-based payment to other forms of care, including ambulatory care. In applying approaches developed for one form of care to another, one must consider whether the same characteristics and conditions apply. This article reviews the similarities and differences between ambulatory and inpatient care in light of available research. It identifies critical issues that should be considered in designing ambulatory payment reform and draws conclusions on the appropriateness of extending case-based payment principles to ambulatory care.

Grimaldi, P. L. Inching toward prospective payment for outpatient hospital care. *Nursing Management* 18(8):26–28, Aug. 1987.

The Health Care Financing Administration (HCFA) has recently revised and expanded the list of ambulatory surgical procedures that Medicare reimburses on a prospective basis. This represents a step toward the federal government's goal of reimbursing all outpatient-hospital care at fixed, predetermined rates. To accommodate this change, hospitals must begin to implement operational changes in medical record documentation, billing, and information system requirements. This article provides information regarding the proposed changes in ambulatory surgery payment as they affect covered procedures and reimbursement. It also discusses impending changes in the system and how they will affect both the ambulatory surgery market and the hospital outpatient area.

Kelly, W., Fillmore, H., and Tenan, P. Case mix classification and ambulatory care. *Business and Health* 5(8):41–44, May 1988.

The Secretary of the Department of Health and Human Services is mandated by Congress to develop prospective payment systems for ambulatory surgery and other outpatient services under Medicare by 1989 and 1991, respectively. Consequently, attention is being focused on adapting one of the many ambulatory care case mix systems being tested across the country. One of these is the products of ambulatory care (PAC) classification system developed under the auspices of the New York State Ambulatory Care Reimbursement Demonstration Project. This article describes the nature of a case mix classification system as it relates to productivity measurement, and then describes and analyzes the PAC system's capabilities to predict resource use and assess quality.

Lutz, S. Changing rules for ambulatory care reimbursement fuel shifts in industry. *Modern Healthcare* 18(26):58–59, July 22, 1988.

Regulatory changes in ambulatory care reimbursement continue to affect the health care industry, although a prospective payment system for all outpatient services is still to come. Owing to a dramatic increase in both outpatient visits and revenue, the federal government is seeking to have an outpatient prospective payment system in place by 1991. This article explores the federal government's initiatives in developing an outpatient prospective payment system, focusing specifically on reimbursement changes that have already been implemented for ambulatory surgery centers, outpatient cancer centers, and outpatient radiological procedures. An examination of reimbursement changes for home care services is also provided.

Schneider, K. C., Lichterstein, J. L., and others. Ambulatory visit groups: an outpatient classification system. *Journal of Ambulatory Care Management* 11(3):1–12, Aug. 1988.

In the late 1970s, researchers at Yale University began developing a system to describe or classify encounters in the ambulatory setting. This article updates the research completed on the ambulatory visit groups (AVG) system and its application to the outpatient service delivery system. It provides information on using AVGs to manage facilities more effectively, define case mix, compare the economic performance of different facilities, and form the basis for a prospective payment system. In addition, information is provided on the objectives of the current AVG study and the guidelines followed in the development of AVGs. The remainder of the article is devoted to describing how AVGs are constructed, focusing on defining major ambulatory diagnostic categories, procedure AVGs, and medical AVGs. In summary, AVGs were developed as a tool to better understand and manage ambulatory health services. Each AVG can be considered to define a product of a health facility.

Young, W. W., Zoyce, D. J., and others. Incorporating the cost of ambulatory care into case-mix-based hospital reimbursement. *Journal of Ambulatory Care Management* 11(3):54–67, Aug. 1988.

The need to categorize inpatient and ambulatory services and to estimate the costs associated with each has become particularly critical in recent years. Implementation of Medicare's prospective payment system (PPS) represents a major step toward encouraging hospitals to examine their mix of patients and services. The system, however, still does not integrate outpatient and inpatient payments. In order to put payment for ambulatory care on the same scale as payment for inpatient care, there is a need for a meaningful way to classify ambulatory services and identify the costs associated with these services. This article describes an ambulatory service classification and cost-weighting system that can be used to integrate inpatient and outpatient payment. The article provides a description of the analytic approach used in the development of this ambulatory service weighting system, examples of the application of the weighting methodology, and a description of the system's strengths and limitations.

Quality Assurance/Risk Management

Anderson, J. G., Benson, D. S., Schweer, H. M., and others. AmbuQual: a computer-supported system for the measurement and evaluation of quality in ambulatory care settings. *Journal of Ambulatory Care Management* 12(1):27–37, Feb. 1989.

> A major impetus for the measurement of quality of care arises from cost-containment effects. Health care providers increasingly are faced with the dilemma of controlling costs without compromising quality. Control of quality, however, requires clear, reliable measures and an information system that measures quality over time and identifies factors that account for variations in quality. This article discusses the development of AmbuQual, an ambulatory care quality assurance system. It provides examples of current methods of quality assurance measurement in the ambulatory setting, analyzes the parameters of ambulatory care that reflect high-quality care and their weighting schemes, and examines the conceptual framework around which AmbuQual was developed.

Benson, D. S., Gartner, C., and others. The ambulatory care parameter: a structured approach to quality assurance in the ambulatory care setting. *QRB* 13(2):51–55, Feb. 1987.

> Ambulatory care parameters are defined by the author as those variables that directly relate to the health of patients. The framework proposed in the article can be used in almost any type of ambulatory care setting; it gives ambulatory health care professionals a means of gaining control of the complexities of ambulatory care. The parameters identified as critical to a successful ambulatory care quality assurance program are practitioner performance, appropriateness of service, patient compliance, support staff performance, accessibility, continuity of care, patient risk minimization, medical record system, patient satisfaction, and cost of services. The article discusses the relevancy of those parameters in monitoring quality of care, the relationship of the parameters to Joint Commission on Accreditation of Healthcare Organi-

zations standards, and the relative value of each parameter. The ambulatory care department of Methodist Hospital in Indianapolis, Indiana, has developed a quality assurance program, called AmbuQual, based on the 10 parameters.

Berman, S. Quality assurance in ambulatory health care. *QRB* 14(1):18–21, Jan. 1988.

This article summarizes the salient issues discussed at the "National Conference on Quality Assurance in Ambulatory Health Care," a symposium sponsored by the Joint Commission on Accreditation of Healthcare Organizations. It gives insights on such issues as employers' concerns about quality of care provided to their employees, consumers' concerns about access to health care and the personal quality of care, organizing an effective quality assurance program, measuring the quality of care, risk management in ambulatory care facilities, and managed care market trends and their impact on quality of care. In addition, the article describes three studies undertaken to study quality assurance in ambulatory health care.

Gonnella, J. S., and Louis, D. Z. Evaluation of ambulatory care. *Journal of Ambulatory Care Management* 11(3):68–83, Aug. 1988.

This article presents an overview of some of the issues involved in assessing the quality of ambulatory care and describes a specific approach—disease staging—as a means of identifying patients who are admitted to hospitals either too early or too late in their disease evolution. It provides an analysis of three predominant approaches to analyzing quality of care: structural, process, and outcome analyses. Factors that contribute to outcomes are also discussed. The remainder of the article focuses on disease-staging methodology, an outcome-based system. The authors define the system, provide examples of the use of disease staging to measure quality of care, and analyze studies of hospitals that have implemented disease staging in evaluating ambulatory care.

Imperato, G. L. An approach to risk management. *Ambulatory Care* 7(7):22–24, July 1987.

A risk management effort in the ambulatory care setting must include what is essentially a readjustment of focus for the entire medical team to one that centers on the patient. A basic understanding must be developed in those on the medical team of the rightful expectations of patients and the need to communicate and interact in ways that foster loyalty, trust, and cooperation. This article provides a brief, succinct overview of the role that risk management programs play in the ambulatory care setting. It discusses medical malpractice litigation, the costs associated with the present medical malpractice crises, keys to developing a functioning risk management plan, factors that act as possible precautions to a malpractice suit, patient expectations of care, and the role physician leadership plays in advancing a successful risk management program.

Palmer, R. H. The challenges and prospects for quality assessment and assurance in ambulatory care. *Inquiry* 25(1):119–31, Spring 1988.

As hospital cost containment has moved care into the ambulatory setting, quality assurance requirements have followed. Because there is neither a uniform ambulatory care data system, nor evidence and expertise on which to base either clinical or management standards for ambulatory care, there are problems in assessment and assurance of quality of ambulatory care. In this article, the author addresses the problems of assessing quality in ambulatory care settings by defining the characteristics of ambulatory care, the dimensions of quality in primary care, the types of data needed to assess quality in primary care, and the standards and criteria needed for quality assessment. The article also provides an analysis of emerging challenges and opportunities, as well as the prerequisites for quality assurance in primary care.

Safranski, P. G., and Safranski, A. J. Getting and keeping medical certification. A quality assurance program for ambulatory surgical centers. *Medical Group Management Journal* 36(2):38–43, 45, Mar.–Apr. 1989.

Getting and keeping medical certification is becoming more challenging every year. It is imperative that the ambulatory surgery center develop and maintain comprehensive documentation to verify compliance with the standards. The surgicenter should also plan for increased interaction with their state's peer review organization in the areas of medical necessity and appropriateness of care.

Wakefield, D. S., and Ludke, R. L. Developing an ambulatory care risk management (ACRM) program. *Journal of Ambulatory Care Management* 11(4):77–87, Nov. 1988.

This article discusses the major issues related to developing ambulatory care risk management (ACRM) programs. The critical differences between inpatient and outpatient models of care are examined, the criteria for assessing potential professional negligence in the ambulatory care setting are discussed, and five areas that need to be considered in developing an ambulatory care risk management program are presented. These areas suggest that providers build on existing inpatient risk management issues and programs, determine adequacy of medical record documentation systems, clarify and document provider and patient responsibilities, evaluate the effects of organizational considerations and financial incentives, and standardize risk assessment of new health care technologies.

Strategic Planning

Cates, N. Entrepreneurial models and applications for hospitals and health-related organizations. *SAM Advanced Management Journal* 26(2):41–46, Summer 1987.

> As a result of a heightened level of competition in the health care marketplace, many hospitals are adopting a business orientation in operating their facility. They now use such business functions as strategic planning, marketing, and sales and advertising. There is increasing emphasis on product line, productivity, cost accounting, and customer orientation. To accommodate this changing environment, many hospitals have elected to use an entrepreneurial strategy—that is, planned innovation built into the organization—to develop modified and new product lines or services. This article identifies and describes models of structured and managed entrepreneurship found in business and industry that can be adopted, perhaps in modified form, by hospitals and other health care organizations. These include the nine-step model, the Detroit Edison Model, the 3M model, the holding company model, and changing the corporate culture.

Cronin, F. J., and Goodspeed, S. W. Beyond strategic planning. *Healthcare Executive* 3(3):28–31, May–June 1988.

> The essence of strategic planning is vision. To classify this vision, health care executives must position their organizations through a step-by-step process. This article describes this process in detail through examining the strategic efforts of Health NorthEast, a not-for-profit hospital holding company. It provides a perspective on the company's decision to redesign the organization for a future purpose, specifically focusing on how they developed strategies that supported both their vision and their mission. Additionally, the article describes the features of Health North-East's new diversified, integrated corporation, the steps they followed in developing a dynamic vision statement, how their new organizational structure supported its mission, and the key strategies selected to fulfill the organization's vision and mission.

Goldstone, A. R. How to establish a medical center. *Journal of Ambulatory Care Marketing* 1(1):47–51, Spring–Summer 1987.

> Setting up an ambulatory care center involves a complex set of procedures and utilizes many different disciplines. This article explores the various decisions that go into establishing and constructing an ambulatory care center. It discusses site location through the use of such market research techniques as assessing demand for the service, competitor analysis, and demographic surveys. It also provides information on choosing a neighborhood for the center and choosing a specific location, such as in a retail shopping center. Other issues discussed in the article include signage and visibility, lease negotiation, purchasing equipment and office supplies, staffing, and advertising.

Markezin, E. T., Katz, G., and Rozenberg, C. Strategic financial planning for ambulatory care services. *Topics in Health Care Financing* 11(4):51–56, Summer 1985.

> Ambulatory care is an area of rapid growth and complex competitive pressures. Real opportunities are available, but the competitive nature of the marketplace inevitably results in some failures. Strategic financial planning to identify optimal directions for new services and to ensure optimal financial results is necessary to successfully compete in the ambulatory care market. Special issues confronting ambulatory care programs are the need to collect reliable and informative data on physician productivity; demand and market penetration and the performance of service units; an understanding of capital needs; the development of organizational structures to accommodate the new programs; and an understanding of product line management. The authors provide a series of applications that used strategic financial planning.

Morris, D. E., and Rau, S. E. Strategic competition: the application of business planning techniques to the hospital marketplace. *Health Care Strategic Management* 3(1):17–20, Jan. 1985.

> Survival in the increasingly turbulent and uncertain health care environment should stimulate the use and application of business planning and corporate strategy techniques. With hospital mergers and acquisitions expected to increase and with cost-containment pressures being exerted by both government and industry, the hospitals that survive will be those that are able to sustain a competitive advantage. The successful players will be those institutions that identify and exploit new opportunities and concentrate management and financial resources in those segments of the market in which competitive advantages are real and attainable.

The article suggests ways to create a strategic focus while still recognizing the barriers and advantages to successful implementation.

Tucker, S. L., and Burr, R. M. Strategic market planning. *Topics in Health Care Financing* 14(3):44–55, Spring 1988.

In today's tumultuous environment, the hospital executive must decide what role the institution will play in the changing medical marketplace. The thoroughness of the decision-making process and the quality of the decisions made are enhanced by appropriate business strategic planning and management tools. This article discusses several of these tools, pointing out their advantages, disadvantages, and overall usefulness in assisting health care decision makers to position their facilities for the future. The strategy tools discussed include the market attractiveness-business positioning planning model, the marketing mix approach, the product line management posture, and the market entry strategy. In addition, the article reviews the essentials behind the financial analysis of the service.

Walker, L. R., and Rosko, M. D. Evaluation of health care service diversification options in health care institutions and programs by portfolio analysis: a marketing approach. *Journal of Health Care Marketing* 8(1):48–59, March 1988.

Originally conceived as a technique to assess how well current activities contribute to the attainment of organizational goals, portfolio analysis can also be used as a market research tool for considering the relative merits of various diversification options under consideration by institutional decision makers. The authors describe the features of portfolio analysis and its use as a tool in the evaluation of health care diversification options. A case study of a hospital that employed this method in its corporate planning and marketing efforts illustrates the use of this analysis technique.

Ziegeler, D. B. Product-line management outside the hospital. *Health Care Strategic Management* 6(2):12–13, Feb. 1988.

This article illustrates how one company applied the theories of product line management to services provided on an outpatient basis. The company, Clinishare, provides preand posthospitalization technologies for all payers and is a for-profit subsidiary of Health West Foundation, a hospital system. Noticing a lack of cohesiveness and synergy among its nine operating units, Clinishare decided to resolve this problem by developing outpatient focus programs, similar to hospital strategic business units. The article illustrates how these focus programs helped the company solve the problem of fragmented posthospital care for diabetics. It also describes the reasons behind the company's acquisition of SugarFree Centers, a supplier of diabetes products, health food, literature, and education and training programs.

Technology

Cowart, R. G., and Freeman, K. M. Mobile high-technology joint ventures. *Journal of Ambulatory Care Management* 11(4):15–22, Nov. 1988.

High-tech, high-ticket equipment is becoming increasingly important in today's health care environment as a means of providing an appropriate standard of care and maintaining an institution's competitive position. High-technology equipment, particularly magnetic resonance imaging (MRI) equipment and lithotripters, carry million-dollar-plus price tags and also frequently involve million-dollar operational budgets. Because many community hospitals and ambulatory care centers cannot individually afford to own and operate such expensive technology, they are increasingly turning to joint ventures to acquire such equipment on a mobile basis, which guarantees utilization and spreads financial risk. This article discusses the cooperative means for achieving a fair arrangement among institutions that establish such joint ventures. It covers such issues as types of mobile high-technology ventures, possible participants, technology selection, medical staff participation, site issues, scheduling, joint venture services, payment considerations, regulatory issues, and tax issues, to name a few.

Dei Rossi, J. A., and Falk, G. Outpatient care technology: problems and opportunities. *Healthcare Executive* 3(6):33–34, Nov.–Dec. 1988.

Payment systems — prospective payment, contracts, and capitation — favor outpatient settings and their lower overhead, although the immediate future in this area is uncertain. The increasing availability of simpler, less costly noninvasive technology and advances in computer components such as microprocessers have helped to shift more inpatient care to the ambulatory care market. This article explores the shift of certain technology from the inpatient to the outpatient market. It gives advice on understanding the forces behind the shift, anticipating the occurrence of this shift, and initiating preemptive measures to slow the rate of change and its impact on inpatient revenue and personnel.

Dougherty, E., and Hagin, D. Mobile lithotripsy services: best bet for most hospitals. *Health Care Strategic Management* 7(3):1, 18–22, Mar. 1989

Now in their third generation, renal lithotripters have become the non-invasive treatment of choice for destroying kidney stones. Extracorporeal shock wave lithotripsy (ESWL) uses high-energy shock waves to pulverize the stones into gravel-like fragments, which a patient usually passes within a few weeks. Buying a million-dollar lithotripter is unlikely to be profitable for the typical community hospital. A machine owned by only one facility will rarely be used at full capacity and will impose an unnecessary financial burden on its owner. Yet hospitals need to provide their patients and physicians with access to state-of-the-art technology, including lithotripsy, to remain competitive. A joint venture or mobile lithotripsy arrangement, not full ownership, is almost always the best strategy. This article explores the idea of mobile lithotripsy units as a means by which hospitals can provide this technology to the communities they serve. It first examines the growth in ESWL, emphasizing factors that are both impeding and promoting growth. It then discusses the advantages and disadvantages of mobile units, joint ventures in lithotripter ownership, the role of specialist input into the development of lithotripter ownership, the role of specialist input into the development of lithotripsy services, and future clinical application of ESWL.

Henderson, J. A. Diagnostic imaging. Can the freestanding center market keep up the pace? *Health Industry Today* 51(2):20–23, Feb. 1988.

Common to all new medical technologies, such as computed tomography (CT) scanning, magnetic resonance imaging, ultrasound, and low-dose mammography, is their capacity for use in either hospital or ambulatory settings. The noninvasive nature of these diagnostic procedures, coupled with increased third-party reimbursement and its cost advantages, have led to a deployment of diagnostic imaging to the outpatient market. This article explores and analyzes the diagnostic imaging market. It describes the various types of imaging centers (hospital-based, freestanding, and mobile), provides national market data that depict their growth and describes centers by type and mix of equipment, and gives market projections. Outpatient diagnostic imaging is now a firmly established reality, and this market can be expected to grow as the demand for diagnostic services expands over the next several years.

New technologies for your hospital to consider. A strategic planning and capital budgeting checklist. *Health Technology* 1(4):138–48, July–Aug. 1987.

This article discusses important new technologies to which hospital CEOs, planners, and clinicians should devote close attention as they plan their capital acquisitions for the future. The article is divided into three sections. The first describes new technologies that both community hospitals and tertiary care centers should consider purchasing, such as gastrointestinal endoscopy and conventional computed tomography (CT), to name a few. Support technologies, such as information systems, home care technologies, and personal emergency response systems, are also discussed. The second section identifies additional technologies that are best described as "emerging." These include such imaging technologies as the high-speed Cine-CT system, photoradiation therapy, gallstone lithotripsy, and hyperthermia for treatment of tumors. The third section of the report describes technologies that should not be considered for acquisition at this time, either because they have not yet demonstrated sufficient clinical effectiveness relative to their cost, or because there is some doubt about their safety.

Planning a pain management program. *Health Technology* 1(3):99–106, May–June 1987.

Pain management programs can be profitable new services. In their planning, hospitals must consider the program's primary approach as well as the therapies to be offered. This article provides information that will prove useful in the preliminary planning of a pain management center. It outlines the operation of pain management programs, provides guidance on staffing, space, and equipment requirements, and discusses the income potential for pain management programs. Depending upon the anticipated patient mix, whether or not local third parties pay for specific therapies may be crucial to program success.

Schmid, G. C., Poulin, M. M., and McNeal, B. R. The impact of new diagnostic technologies on health care. An aggregation of expert opinion. *Journal of Health Care Technology* 2(3):167–82, Winter 1986.

The growing number of applications for both new and existing technologies will act as a catalyst for major changes in the diagnostic testing field in the 1990s. This article summarizes the results of a study undertaken by the Institute for the Future (IFTF) to identify the technologies that are likely to have great impact on the diagnostic testing market and to document forthcoming changes in the location, type, and cost of diagnostic testing. Specifically, it reports on the major environmental factors affecting the industry, future diagnostic technologies, market impacts, and implications of these changes for the character and environment of the diagnostic market.

Sprague, G. R. Managing technology assessment and acquisition. *Healthcare Executive* 3(6):26–29, Nov.–Dec. 1988.

To remain competitive in the ever-changing health care marketplace, health care executives must make critical decisions about the allocation of capital for the purchase of high-technology medical equipment. However, sometimes these serious capital commitment decisions are made with limited financial and clinical data. This article provides the health care executive with information that will guide and support capital investment decisions. It specifically points out the need to develop ongoing technology assessment committees; involve physicians in the technology assessment process; consider new options in allocating resources; establish strategic and financial priorities and balance the use of resources with goals through innovative financing; coordinate facility planning, design, and construction; take charge of the acquisition process; and maintain the advantage over the vendor when going operational.

Wilkinson, R. New technology that will change key services. *Hospitals* 62(10):56–61, May 20, 1988.

Medical researchers, technology experts, and analysts were interviewed to identify key developments in the areas of cardiology, oncology, women's health, orthopedics, and neurology. These five areas were identified by CEOs as ripe for future product line growth and development. For each of the five areas, the article summarizes how future technology will shape medical management of diseases, reduce the cost of treatment, move more procedures to the outpatient setting, and assist physicians in diagnosing diseases earlier than in the past. It also discusses the role management will play in integrating new technology into both the organization and the patient care process.